IT'S NOT WEIRD ANYMORE

AN EXTRAORDINARY TRUE TALE

BY LAURA LEGERE

An entertaining educational adventurous self-help resource guide to
spiritual and health wisdom, conspiracy, sacred sex and a Match.com
love relationship.

IT'S NOT WEIRD ANYMORE

AN EXTRAORDINARY TRUE TALE

BY LAURA LEGERE

An entertaining educational adventurous self-help resource guide to spiritual and health wisdom, conspiracy, sacred sex and a Match.com love relationship.

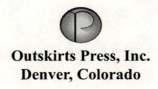

Outskirts Press, Inc.
Denver, Colorado

~ Dedication ~

This book is dedicated to Peter and Julie and my incredible family, friends, their family and friends, my visible and invisible angels, and all my amazing teachers and healers. It's Not Weird Anymore is a tribute to all of you. Thank you for your genuine contribution in my life.

Here's to Your Awakened Metamorphosis, Love, Light, and Freedom,

Laura Legere

Table of Contents

It's Not Weird Anymore is an eclectic soup of a love story, Match. com, relationship, sacred sex, natural healing methods, essential oils, sound health advice, personal growth, metaphysical magick, archetypes, art, belly dancing, feng shui, spirit, wisdom, politics, and conspiracy spun together as an entertaining self-help teaching tool.

~ About the Author ~

Laura Legere's focus of service and purpose is assisting people with healthy living, personal growth, and spiritual exploration through her private practice as a massage therapist and teacher of natural healing in essential oils. She has always been a gifted networker as well as a great storyteller and loves to point people in a purposeful, positive direction.

~ Disclaimer ~

Everything written in this book is my opinion and experience and I am sure there are those who would disagree. If you do anything I suggest without the supervision of a licensed medical doctor who generally knows very little about natural health solutions, you do so at your own risk. Medical doctors play a vital role especially when it comes to necessary trauma surgery and I am very fortunate to be here in this day and age when surgeons have amazing skills. The publisher and the author, the distributors and bookstores, present this information for educational purposes only. I am not making an attempt to prescribe any medical treatment, since under the laws of the United States only a licensed medical doctor (an MD) can do so. You and only you are responsible if you choose to do anything based on what you read.

Laura Legere

~ Foreword ~

Laura is one of a kind and you are about to embark into her interpersonal world of heart, soul, and consciousness. I knew we would become friends for life when we met belly dancing back in 1996, in Maui, Hawaii. Forty-two dancers shimmering, sensuous, alive, feminine goddesses all together under the wings of Delilah, our most cherished belly dance teacher. Learning undulations at the ocean's edge, calling us to move our hips and pelvis into her warm, salty, wild embrace. We performed sacred ritual dances into the Maui Sea, in the early morning hours with the sunrise and laughed, frolicked, and danced until our hearts were satisfied and our souls were dripping in the divine joy of the Goddess.

Laura and I would stay awake into the wee hours of the night reminiscing about the ancient days of Egypt, the men in our lives, politics, and our committed path to uplift the weary ones longing to remember who we truly are, including ourselves.

We healers have a different life, an unusual path, and a purpose that is bigger than we know or can comprehend at times. I have been privileged to watch and witness Laura grow and change and become a magnificent being of such grace. Has it always been easy? No. Has it all been worth it? YES! Are we still standing? Of course we are, because we have each other to bounce ideas off of and share the most intimate details of our forever evolving lives. One thing about Laura that stands out is how she embraced some profoundly deep teachings of consciousness that she will share with you in the upcoming pages.

We all go through lessons in life and some we file away in an intellectual manner and if we are wise, we take new pearls of wisdom and embody them, call them our own, and become that which we embraced. Laura is a profound receptacle for this and I have watched her grow into a remarkable, powerful, wise woman who is self-empowered, caring, loving, alive, and beautiful.

I was with Laura and her crazy, intense incident in Mexico. I watched her warrior come forth like I had never seen before. I saw her apply her new lessons to a most difficult and challenging circumstance. I observed her go through it in a way that is forever imprinted on my own soul and carried me through many storms of my own.

In the pages that follow, read what she shares with a mind that is open, free from opinion, and if you are so moved, begin to embrace your own feminine warrior. Laura is a profound and important mirror for us all.

In Joy

Julie Chertow

~ Introduction ~

I felt compelled to write this book in honor of all the wonderful people doing amazing service work on the planet and how I have benefited. This book is a tribute to all of you and to the readers seeking this information.

It's Not Weird Anymore serves as an entertaining, educational health advice, personal growth, spiritual love story, and a detailed self-help resource directory. I did not want to weigh the story down with details about the many methods, techniques, and programs that are introduced in the narrative. The resource section is designed to cover these details so you can flip back and forth and read about them when you desire, or wait until the end of the story.

The resource directory is entertaining as well, with interesting wisdom, knowledge, and commentary. Some of the commentary is about events that happened after the story was finished. I chose not to put websites all over the book and instead have a central website with links to all of the resources there. There are extra resources in the directory that are not in the story; whatever helps people is in there. You will find everything linked in the book and more at: *www.ItsNotWeirdAnymore.com.* Be sure to use this username: *itsnotweirdanymore* and this password: *iamlove* to gain access. Please use your intuition and discernment when doing your own research on the Internet. I have found intentional misinformation written on the Internet about the teachers and programs many others and I have benefitted from.

Read with a relaxed open heart and mind and enjoy the wild ride!

It's Not Weird Anymore

*An entertaining, educational, adventurous self-help resource
guide to spiritual and health wisdom, conspiracy, sacred sex,
and a Match.com love relationship.*

An extraordinary true tale by Laura Legere

~ 1 ~

Julie was in front of me as she guided my way on her scooter while I followed
close behind on mine. The hot Mexican weather with the crystal blue ocean and
its breeze felt perfect on our exposed skin while the cruise ship waited for our
return to sail back to the states from Cozumel. The road had turned rough and we
decided to turn around and get back to a smooth surface and feel safe again. As
we sped our way on new asphalt, I followed Julie around a long, slow curve to the
left and instead of following the curve I kept going straight, all the while thinking,
Why would I do this, it makes no sense, this can't be good. My scooter crashed
into the rocks and I flew over the handlebars and landed face first into a coral
rock. I immediately pulled my face off the rock and felt the bones in my upper
jaw floating around and a large gap where I thought my front teeth should be. My
first thought was, *I am going to start bleeding and have a hell of a headache.* The
bleeding started as I stood up and began to climb out of the shallow, solid rock
ditch. Julie had turned around as she witnessed my mistake in her rearview mirror
and waited across the street for traffic to clear.

"Are you okay?" she asked.

"No," I said.

Just then a man walked up to me and said,

"I'm a doctor."

I thought, *Well, that's good 'cause I could sure use one right now.* He sat me down, instructed me to open my eyes, and checked them while he asked a few questions that I could easily answer. With Julie by my side she asked him what could she do? He requested something to soak the blood and she pulled out two large beach towels from my backpack that we brought from the cruise ship. He told me I would be all right and he handed me over to the ambulance that happened to be close by.

My right eye was beginning to swell shut and the image imprinted in my mind while my left eye began to close was a small Mexican EMT looking over my head to Julie, whispering,

"Don't worry."

Everything went dark as I stayed awake and felt the small Mexican EMTs move my body onto the stretcher. I could hear them say,

"Uno, dos, tres, huh."

My 5' 9" muscular body was a giant to them. This was humorous to me and I giggled to myself. As the ambulance cruised toward the Cozumel Medical Center Hospital I mentioned to Julie what I thought happened in my mouth.

"I think I lost my front teeth and shoved the rest of them up into the roof of my mouth."

Julie told me later that she did not want to hear that since she was holding my nose on at that point. We both got quiet and began to chant devotional Tibetan silently to ourselves to shift the energy. I chanted, *Nam Myoho Renge Kyo.* Julie confessed later that she chanted, *Nam Myoho Renge Kyo, Fuck! Nam Myoho Renge Kyo, Fuck!*

During the journey to the hospital I was asked several times what my name and age were and I could always answer correctly.

"Laura Legere, fifty-one."

When we arrived the doctors put me through every X-ray machine they had and this took what seemed like hours. At some point someone squeezed my nose and it felt like crepe paper. I could tell they were assessing the extent of the damage and I hoped they would be done soon so I could go back to the ship. I was told I would not be going back to the ship and a few minutes later advised I could not fly home either. I asked about all my belongings on the ship and was told that Julie went to fetch everything and would stay with me. I thought about Peter, my brand-new boyfriend, who was just moving in with me while I went on this cruise with Julie. My thoughts were, *I stayed alive for him too.* There was no doubt in my mind that he would still pursue our relationship despite the situation. I continued to chant silently and noticed I had not experienced any pain, not even a headache. I never even experienced pain on impact. I tuned into my body and felt grateful that I kept myself so healthy and could feel my body's systems performing their job in the healing process.

After the examination was finished it was determined that I had no cervical damage and I did not lose any teeth. I had broken my whole face. The right orbital bone (right eye) was broken and swollen shut; my upper palate broke in half and caused the gap between my front teeth. My long Native American nose with a ridge was flattened and half off on the right side. The sinus bones were broken along with my upper gum and cheekbones in places. We would have to wait and see if I could see out of my right eye when the swelling was down enough to open it.

I was wheeled into a curtained area in a hallway and got prepped for nose surgery. Apparently I needed a nose immediately and in the meantime Julie was frantically taking care of everything.

I waited silently for the surgeon and kept the chant going in my head. I finally had to pee and asked for my very first bedpan. That was strange; I tried lying flat at first and felt it was not going to happen that way, so I sat up and did it and felt much better.

Julie came around to discuss the $400 cash deductible for the scooter. The scooter company sent two employees who sat at the hospital for three hours waiting for Julie to give them their money. She asked them about the insurance we bought to ride the scooters and they replied that they would have covered my accident if I had gone to the other hospital. Julie and I were both too weary and had too many other things to deal with than to contest their ridiculous claim. I told Julie where the cash was to pay them and she said they appeared happy to go home and forget about us.

I told Julie where my phone book was so she could call my family. She had called Peter earlier in the afternoon and left a message. He was in his first day of a three-day Aromatherapy Intensive I recommended and had his phone turned off. It was evening by now so Julie called my sister Ruth first. Ruth was very emotional and upset, and so were many of my family and friends. Julie gave me the phone to speak to Ruth and she was glad I could talk coherently to her. I mentioned the positive things, like I didn't lose any teeth and I was exceedingly happy about that. I asked her to call Peter and tell him I love him and that I am normally a low-maintenance girlfriend. We laughed and that helped lighten up the situation a little. I am so used to being the healer and helping others with their comfort that this was quite a different experience. All of my personal growth programs were tested to the max on this one and a particular one came to mind, PGP (Personal Growth Program). My PGP coaches kept me on my toes with their deep, penetrating questions that I would never think to ask myself. This program has shown me how much I chose to suffer about my choices and circumstances. I remained very conscious lying in my Mexican hospital bed to not suffer about my situation, just stay in the present, take care of business, and keep my mind clear. I hypothesize that this is one of the major reasons I did not suffer from any physical pain whatsoever. One doctor thought I did not understand how severe my injuries were because I wasn't freaking out and just remained calm.

IT'S NOT WEIRD ANYMORE

~ 2 ~

I have had a theory for a long time that we tend to make an injury worse with our minds than the actual physical damage that happened in the first place. Some people can have the same exact injury and one will completely recover as if nothing had happened and the other person will hold on to that old injury for the rest of their life. I observed this behavior when I worked at a blue-collar job with the city for seven years. In my opinion it shows the degree we choose to suffer. I was able to test my theory on myself years ago when I threw my hip out in belly dance class. It came out of its socket; boy did that hurt! My fellow belly-dancing friends guided me to the floor and handed me a popsicle to recover while I watched them finish the class. I was lifted up to stand and found I could not walk forward, so my dancing healer friends drove my car and my sore body home and put me to bed. They said they would pick me up in the morning and take me to their Shiatsu practitioner. My boyfriend at the time came to spend the night, because I could not get to the bathroom on my own. He had to literally drag me to the toilet in the middle of the night.

In the morning my friends showed up as they said they would and drove me to the Shiatsu practitioner. They practically carried me in, because I could not walk yet. He instructed me to put on a little white plastic gown, just like in a clinic. I told him what my problem was and he motioned for me to lie on the table. He started working his way through my meridians (major nerves and arteries) with his lean, small stature and enormously muscular arms. Every time he tightly held the acupressure points it was painful, but I could feel massive amounts of energy move through my body and out my feet. Sometimes he held me so tight in places I would grab his arms and try to pull them off. Unusual behavior for me since I was a massage therapist. It felt like he was chasing me around the table and then he grabbed my sore hip as I belted out,

"That's my hip!"

"You'll be alright," he said and gave a loud laugh.

When he finished the 30-minute session he told me that I would begin walking straight without a limp within 24 hours and to be conscious not to limp after that. He also said to continue to work on my massage clients and not lie around thinking I was recovering; that would make it worse. I paid him $30 and was able to walk out of his office. I stuck to his advice and tested out my theory. Within 24 hours I did not have a limp, started a yoga immersion (yoga every morning at 6 a.m. for 30 days straight), and never missed a belly dance class. I felt some soreness, but that was all and within three weeks I could not tell I had injured anything.

~ 3 ~

I believe my theory especially applies to the more current situation at hand in the Cozumel Medical Center.

Soon the surgeon and his helpers came to put my nose back on. He administered the numbing agent all around my cheeks and mouth and began re-building and sewing my nose back together. I continued to silently chant and changed the chant to *Om Mani Padme Hum.* As Dr. Morales began to sew the right side of my nose back on I could feel the thread moving through the skin without any pain. The project went on for over two hours; at the end he packed my nose completely and it stayed that way for five days.

My doctors said they had contacted the best plastic surgeon in all of Mexico and he was prepared to fly from Mexico City and perform the reconstruction or resurrection or restoration, whichever you prefer, surgery. My family and Julie were worried about me being in another country and having surgery. They wanted to check on the air ambulance situation because I could not fly economy in my condition, especially with broken sinuses.

After the nose surgery was finished I sat up and started talking to Julie. She was so glad to see and hear me speaking. She began to tell me how she was starting to feel relief as the support from our family and friends comforted her after feeling so stressed and overwhelmed. She explained how she had five minutes to pack both of our suitcases and get off the ship after the accident. Cruise ships do not wait for anyone. She said there were about 14 people in our stateroom helping throw our stuff in the suitcases and as soon as she stepped off the boat the cruise ship moved away from the loading ramp and was on its way that instant.

I felt so fortunate that she was the one with me in this situation. Julie is an amazing, skilled healer and has influenced my own practice in many ways. To put it simply we are both massage therapists and met at Delilah's Belly Dance Retreat on Maui in 1995 where we became fast friends.

~ 4 ~

Julie and I decided we were platonically married to each other a few years back when the dating scene appeared bleak to us at the time. So we speak to each other the way we desire a divine lover/partner to address us. As a result we call each other *Wifey* and let all our potential mates know we come with a wife. This is our playful humor that means we are the best of friends; we back each other up, will always be a consistent, steady presence no matter what happens with our male relationships, and we check out our potential male partners for each other.

Julie and I have been studying the practice and medicinal use of essential oils since 1996 with Gary Young, creator and CEO of Young Living Essential Oils. We both teach the practical, everyday use of essential oils and I thank Mother/

IT'S NOT WEIRD ANYMORE

Father God for this as our essential oil skills totally prepared us for what was in front and ahead of us. Our reward for being good little essential oil educators and business builders with the company was winning a cruise with 300 other Young Living Essential Oilers. It was our last day on land before heading back to Galveston, Texas, where we originally boarded the ship. It was January 18th, 2007; we rented scooters, went to the beach to snorkel, tan, and do some spiritual work at the Mayan ruins, and on the way back to the ship I went off the road on the scooter.

Julie and I live 600 miles apart—she lives in Ashland, Oregon and I in Seattle, Washington—and we use Young Living business as a way to get together. We usually meet at the yearly conventions, but this time the cruise was a wonderful surprise for us to have a real vacation together. We always take lots of pictures of each other because we wear our finest clothes and always look our best at these events. Julie started taking pictures of me soon after we unpacked. I was sitting on my bed relaxing while she took a head shot of me. I heard her gasp, so I leaned over to see what she was looking at. The picture showed me looking in two directions at once and I looked like a ghost. A double exposure on a digital camera is pretty hard if almost impossible to do, but there it was. We both wondered what that was all about and thought it was weird. Little did we know what lay ahead, and the picture wasn't weird, but a sign along the way.

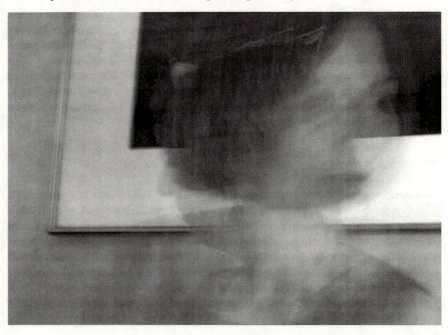

We soon forgot about the picture and had a blast making the most of the cruise. Dune buggy riding in Belize, swimming with dolphins in Honduras, rain forest zip-lining and river cave tubing. Julie and I ended up rescuing two women cave tubing as the strong current pushed them up against the cave wall and de-tubed one of them. Out of 300 Young Living cruisers Julie won a dinner for two with Gary and Mary Young. She invited me to accompany her and I was more than willing and excited to be her guest. At the dinner Mary Young seemed to study my face to the point that I became uncomfortable, and looking back, I think she is very psychic and picked up on my face change, unconsciously of course.

Julie and I ate incredible food, drank our late night cappuccino so we could stay awake dancing in the Sky Lounge for hours, melting the calories away every night. I did not want to come home with extra weight as my new romantic partner Peter was waiting for my return and I wanted to keep looking my best for him and me. I know people can gain a lot of weight on these cruises and with the food availability it's like being placed in front of a delectable pig trough.

~ 5 ~

I was resting in my hospital room with Julie/Wifey in the bed next to me. The hospital staff gave her a bed, changed her sheets and towels, and fed her. We had a bathroom with a shower and greatly appreciated all of this, especially because we knew we would never have experienced this in the United States. The nursing staff was very attentive and checked on me frequently. It appeared as if little dolls were caring for me because they were all extraordinarily beautiful, young, and very small in stature. In the meantime Wifey applied the therapeutic medicinal essential oils directly onto my face that studies have shown can help bring the swelling down, repair the skin, nerves, and bone. Lavender may help with scarring, pain, and nervous tension; frankincense can help boost the immune system, relax muscles, and decrease inflammation and depression, and juniper can help nerve repair, release toxins, increase circulation, work as an antiseptic, and release fluid retention. These oils worked wonders for me, while Julie witnessed the swelling recede 80% in two days. The oils have been proven to be great for fighting infection; therefore I was never at risk of infection, which can often happen during a hospital stay.

I have taken a moment here to convey what I consider important foundational knowledge about the oils. There is a tremendous difference between "100% pure essential oils" and "therapeutic grade essential oils." Essential oils are not regulated in this country, so the labeling does not have much meaning because companies put whatever they want on the label. There are several companies that make strictly synthetic essential oils that have no medicinal qualities and can be dangerous when applied and diffused. The oils mentioned in my healing process are of the highest quality. They are grown in organic fields, harvested in the precise season with the moon cycles, and steam-distilled at the lowest temperatures for an extended amount of time to carry the maximum natural chemical compounds for quick, beneficial results. Many companies will distill their plants for a very short period at high temperatures or dilute with synthetics to make a large quantity quickly. This ruins the medicinal quality and renders them much less effective and dangerous. Other companies chemically extract the oils, making them lose potency as well. I give thanks to Gary Young time and time again for teaching me to be my own healer and making his plant extracts so powerful. The resource section in the back of this book has more detailed information under *Young Living Essential Oils*. Okay, enough health advice for now, back to the Mexican hospital room.

While I rested I heard Julie talking to Peter and I tried to imagine what must be going through his mind, although I knew deep down inside he would not abandon me even though it was only three weeks into our relationship. He had just finished the first full day of a three-day Aromatherapy Intensive. One of the first things I remember saying to him after being handed the phone was,

"It's very important that you stay and finish that class, so you know how to heal me."

He seemed surprised because he was ready to receive instructions on how to be by my side right away. At this point we were not sure if I was staying in Cozumel or flying home on the air ambulance, so he had to stay put for now.

Julie had asked Peter what he was going to do since this was the beginning of our relationship. He replied,

"I will do whatever it takes to help her heal."

"That's good, 'cause most guys would walk away from something like this, especially so early in a relationship," Wifey said.

Wifey and I knew then that I had landed a good one.

Peter mentioned when my sister called to give him the news about my accident, she challenged him and asked how he was going to deal with my face so messed up.

"I didn't fall in love with her face," he told her.

My thought was…*That's right, Peter, show us what you're made of and get to know my family and friends this instant!*

While I continued talking to Peter I gave him all the phone numbers of clients and friends I had scheduled appointments and get-togethers with, so he could let them know I would not be able to meet them. This also spread the word about my situation and people began to concentrate their focus and pray for me. I could literally feel the healing energy being directed toward me.

~ 6 ~

Peter and I met on Match.com in November of 2006. Our profiles matched by 95%, which is very unusual. When your matches are emailed to you they usually match between 68 to 78%. The 5% distinction between our profiles was the distance. He lived in Boise, Idaho and I live in Seattle. I was looking for someone within 25 miles and he expanded his scope to 500 miles.

My profile title read like this:

Health Conscious, Humorous, Deeply Spiritual, Passionate, Adventurous, Personal Growth Oriented Woman

I had been Match.com dating the fall of 2006 and was having fun practicing dating while I observed my date's behavior and myself with my PGP (Personal Growth Program) perspective. I broke through a barrier back in August of 2006 when I watched the movie *The Secret*. It was about how the universe is listening to our inner focus and not what we try to hide in outward appearances. Our constant inner dialogue and focus are what create our personal world of experiences. It's not that this information was new to me, but it put me in touch with what I was really thinking about men and relationships. Here I am on the Internet asking for a relationship and thinking, *I never go out on a second date from the Internet; men cannot challenge me enough; they're too immature; they think I am too weird; all the good ones are taken.* I had an epiphany after watching *The Secret* that if I wanted a relationship with someone who matched my vibration, I had better change my inner dialogue. Surely I was keeping them away from me with my real thoughts, not my affirmations or my profile ad. Your inner dialogue creates your outer world, so what are we thinking? I believe if we have been single for a long time we can create/project a pretty unrealistic view of our future partner. The computer-dating scene in my view can make this an even bigger delusion, because you are not initially interacting with people physically. This makes it easier to stay in fantasy when you read someone's profile as well as his or her emails and even talking on the phone. I think our tendency is to project who we would like to be, and our actions don't necessarily match our words. The other tendency is to project our fantasy/filter onto the other. I believe we all do this, computer or no, but the computer makes it more exaggerated in my opinion. I have found personal growth classes, workshops, seminars, and coaching to be the best choice for clearing yourself and interacting with others in a more realistic way. Self-awareness is very attractive.

When I decided to change my perspective I removed my profile from Tantra. com that had been up for a year, because it's like real estate, when your house has been on the market too long you have fewer prospects. I opened a new profile on Match.com and changed my inner dialogue to *I am surrounded by men and women who connect and introduce me to wide-awake, available men.* I also made a decision to stop looking for the "One" and just "Be One" with whomever I was with. This was much more relaxing, fun, and sexy. I even went out on more than one date with the same person from the Internet. I was enjoying this new way of being while I dated a couple of men for a short time before Peter appeared.

On my profile page I requested a mature, creative goof and the many other attributes I believe I personify. One of the statements in my profile that stood out to Peter was I welcomed constructive feedback and owned my own emotional shortcomings. As I mentioned earlier I enrolled in a personal growth program called PGP that helps clear old negative behavior patterns and works amazingly well. He was also drawn to one of my pictures that showed me standing next to an Egyptian sarcophagus. Most of my closest friends feel a strong Egyptian connection and Peter definitely has that connection too. His profile spoke to me as well, and that mischievous, asking-for-trouble grin in his picture really turned me on. His profile title was *Divine Love*. When he called me for the first time his voice sounded familiar, with his beautiful southern accent, and he said my voice sounded familiar too. I asked him where he was from and he said Bedford, Virginia. I said I was from Roanoke, Virginia and in my excitement I dropped the phone to the floor. Roanoke is 30 miles from Bedford. We laughed and seemed to hit it off right away. He happened to be living in Boise on his brother's horse ranch after a relationship breakup in Florida. His brother had bugged him for years to move out west. Peter had only been living in Boise about five months and was not settled in yet. He had retired from Verizon Telephone Company and could live wherever he chose. For the next month we got to know each other over the phone and email. He would write the most beautiful, spiritual, poetic emails, and I would send him articles and excerpts from David Deida books on the new relationships. David Deida writes and teaches very profound work on our behavior patterns in our masculine/feminine relationships and how to understand and communicate on a deeper level. This gave us much to discuss in our lively conversations, as I had stopped reading David Deida books because I was frustrated about not meeting someone I could relate to on that level. Peter met me on my spiritual and personal growth responsibility level in our conversations, so much so that I didn't have to explain myself very much.

With David Deida's permission I have included the articles and excerpts from his books I sent Peter in the resource section under *Relationship Awakening*. These articles have been circulating the Internet for many years. My online dating profile sold many Deida books, as I received emails from men all over the country requesting more information. They would thank me for turning them onto his material and let me know it held great value and insight for them. I sent Peter personal emails too, but mine were short, brief, and not that interesting; I preferred the phone. Writing this book has challenged me to dig down deeper inside myself, as I am naturally brief and to the point, and a book demands much more detail. Here is my interpretation of the foundation of Deida's work called the *Three Stages of Relationships*.

Note: Deida clarifies in the introduction to his books that the masculine and feminine are energies and do not necessarily mean a man and a woman. He states for the sake of time he does not mention every possible kind of intimate relationship there is. Please read it the way it applies to your particular circumstances. In general women have a tendency to have a greater percentage of a feminine essence and men tend toward a higher percentage of a masculine essence. The distinction between the masculine and feminine essences causes the strong physical attraction.

I believe Deida's description of each stage—first *Dependence*, second *50/50*, and third *Intimate Communion*—are great insight tools to open, expand, and grow through our current relationships. He encourages us to explore our intimacy patterns with an open heart and loving humor.

The *Dependence Relationship* is about power over another and mistaking it for love. The typical old stereotype would be the macho husband and the submissive housewife. One partner needs to feel in control while the other one gives up their authentic power in order to feel loved and accepted. I personally experienced giving up my potency in my first marriage and left because I grew out of it.

The *50/50 Relationship* is about safe boundaries and equal expectations between partners. This is the next step in evolution from the *Dependence Relationship*. This style of relationship is based on two independent individuals with their own source of income negotiating the household chores and bills, etc. This kind of arrangement causes the individual partners to strike their own inner balance between masculine and feminine at home and in the workplace. The *50/50 Relationship* tends to neutralize the masculine/feminine polarities that cause the strong sexual attraction between partners. The fiery passion dissipates and a more brotherly, sisterly, business relationship takes hold. Deep down, the partners may feel incomplete as their sexual essence is suppressed and they yearn to be touched much more deeply than a *50/50 Relationship* offers.

Intimate Communion is feeling safe to let go of cautious boundaries and passionately ravish our partner with delicious, sensual love. We gift our partner with uninhibited, free love, flowing directly from our sexual essence without fear or doubt. According to Deida, love is something you practice, not something you fall in and out of. Love is like practicing the piano or playing tennis, not something you feel or not. In *Intimate Communion* we practice loving through our partner's anger and hurt by moving toward them with an open heart. We learn to love from our deepest core, which comes from the root of our sexual essence.

The complete articles and excerpts of David Deida's are quite long and may take you further away from the story than you may want to go at this point. You have the option of reading them now or later. The titles and pages are:

The Three Stages of Relationships – pages 180 - 181
How the Feminine Grows – pages 182 - 185
Fear and Love – pages 185 - 188
What Men Wish Women Knew – pages 188 - 192
Deviations of the Feminine Heart – pages 192 - 195
Orgasmic Love – pages 195 – 198

IT'S NOT WEIRD ANYMORE

Here are a few emails I saved from Peter, complete with or without punctuation, continuing thoughts in long sentences. The first one is referring to my sending him the David Deida articles and accidentally sending them to someone else's email:

Hi Love,

At least someone else got the blessing of this material. I don't see how someone can be offended by the truth even though I see it all the time. I used to think I was abnormal in high school because guys would talk about girls in ways that seemed so totally unfeeling from where I was experiencing love and relationship or what that should look like. Finally, I resigned myself to the fact that there was no one who could understand even this grander form of surrender into love that seemed to permeate my very soul. It was not until 6 yrs ago or so that I realized that there were others who were seeing the same dream and realization that indeed this is our destiny as man and woman, channels for the divine masculine to flow through and into the divine feminine the total surrender into ultimate bliss. Now I have been thoroughly prepared for the one who is not afraid to walk into this kind of relationship, to be with the one who realizes that the relationships before can now be seen for what they were and be left behind like a cocoon to emerge into this beautiful creature of flight. The more you show me the more my vibrational level goes up and it seems dating anyone else until I meet you is only another lesson in the superficial. How much joy I'm feeling just knowing you are out there and there is this possibility of experiencing what I have always seen in my heart and mind's eye. I don't want to seem like I'm coming on too strong, but how strong do you think the love of all the Cosmos flows when allowed to be freely accepted. There have been those who thought that yes this is what they wanted only to say later (for real) that they couldn't accept this much goodness in their life, or got scared because in the surrender you feel you have lost all control (the choice-less choice) the total giving up into love without concern for self only the adoring and the adored. There is no ego in the way of my loving now, it has burnt away now, for there is no room for it in the face of what I truly am, love itself. Wow I just burned out my broadband connection, hope I can get this thru.

Namaste indeed with all the love and blessings that means, Peter

Over the phone he liked to sing to me from his large collection of classic rock songs, any lyrics that pertained to our coming together. I loved that he could let loose and be uninhibited right off the bat like that.

Hi love of my life,

I was just rereading what a man wants in a woman. In it Deida talks about being in a place where both are open to love completely; I believe he calls it risky business. It's kind of like what you said you were looking for in a man, that the only one who can love with you, as you know it can be experienced, is someone who has reached the same level of spiritual understanding as trust and letting go are beyond what most can even imagine. Seeing myself as a heart true man the email on ho'oponopono really struck me with all kinds of meaning. Healing and addressing all of life that is showing up in one's awareness surely leaves that person more purely open to intimate relationship with another. In this space you realize that there are few who can even come close to being able to live a sacred love with you in all its completeness. You are not willing to settle for anything less because you cannot go back to the previous stages nor being pure love do you have any need to do so. And so it is I who comes offering my truest most divine self to you for there is no one even close to what I am receiving that you are. Truly I am excited as never before and in that I am laying myself wide open, it is the only thing I can do! Ah to freely dissolve one into the other, to play in that realm of adoration.

Love and Blessing Already in All Ways, Peter

Ho'oponopono, which Peter mentions in his email above, is a Hawaiian Shamanic practice of love and forgiveness, way beyond our "normal" understanding. A detailed article of this beautiful practice by Dr. Joe Vitale is in the resource section under *Ho'oponopono.*

Hi love,

Isn't it nice how if you are studying one thing and get material that is covering another area and the two seem to merge and complement each other? The work I have been doing studying Ken Wilber's Integral life/Spirituality show how many truths fit inside each other in levels of awareness that because you come to a higher truth doesn't mean you totally abandon what went before. It seems Deida is trying to show how a man can be feeling, intuitive, and spiritual and still have that masculine drive to have heart and spine. I have felt somehow that I needed to apologize at workshops for being a spiritualist who can go out and enjoy hunting or fishing or enjoys ravishing the woman in my life to enjoy the sensual nature of all this relative world. Deida even makes the comment about being able to be in our pain to not deny or feel guilty that we as men are feeling these feelings as a superior man does not run from such issues but embraces, expresses and then lets go! I see now why you made the statement about choosing to be with a man who can express his discomfort. God how I love you for all you have already given to me, for opening yourself to the possibility of being ravished by a Virginia Scorpio!!! That you are open to examining your truths and changing them as logic and reason of a higher mind/soul dictate. One of my teachers, Andrew Cohen, is in constant evolution and is not stuck in his ego so that he feels he has to stay in what he believed to be true yesterday.

IT'S NOT WEIRD ANYMORE

I have thanked him on several occasions for being bold enough to constantly being available to embrace new truths. Deida talks about the masculine error to think that somewhere down the road is the finish line (I personally feel this is a human condition) when the truth is to be in the creative challenge being in the ongoing tussle, play and making love to all of it with complete abandon knowing life in that type of walk only gets better!!!!!!! Well got to get ready to be the hunter and walk and make love to these beautiful mountains in Oregon where we go. Love hugs and Kisses til we meet, Peter

One of the many profound subjects we talked about was a spiritual community in Northern Italy called Damanhur. He mentioned something about it first, and I chimed in,

"Isn't that the place where they built temples inside of a mountain?"

"Yes," he replied.

He said he traveled there twice, once on an eight-day retreat to Damanhur and another passing through on his way from Egypt and then to India. I was told about Damanhur in one of my metaphysical classes I taught in Roanoke a few years ago by one of my students. When I mentioned this to Peter, he asked for a description of the person and we found that she was on his first trip to Damanhur. I have been fascinated with the place ever since it was described to me and loved listening to Peter talk about his experience there. Damanhur is described in more detail further along in the story.

The more we talked the more we found we knew some of the same people from Virginia. He hung out in the same neighborhood that my mom and I have when I visit her. He owns part of a duplex eight blocks from my mom's house. I have been a friend of Peter's ex's boyfriend before she began her relationship with Peter. The connections kept going on and on. We both worked blue-collar jobs for our livelihoods, he spliced phone fiber-optic cable and I spliced high-voltage cable for the local power company before I started my own business. It's interesting how destiny appears to be at play here and not weird coincidences. Peter and I concluded that we had been dancing around each other for years and never formally met.

I wanted to introduce Peter to Wifey and another friend, Cynthia, and had them check out his profile. They both emailed him personally and introduced themselves as dear friends of mine. They both wrote glowing accounts of our friendship and gave him their Goddess seal of approval. That meant a lot to me and Peter was exhilarated by receiving emails from two beautiful Goddesses welcoming him. Wifey and Peter exchanged several emails and became friends over the computer. Little did they know how much I would need them both a few weeks later.

Here are Wifey and Peter's correspondence emails:

LAURA LEGERE

Dear Divine Love,

Sorry I do not know your name but I am Julie, Laura's Wifey. I know, I know you're thinking this woman I am interested in has a wife? Oh what am I getting myself into?

Well, you see after many disappointments in male/female relationships.... All of my girlfriends agree including Laura that if we could just meet a guy like our girlfriends, that would be amazing! So on that note, Laura and I said well let's get married. So we are plutonic Wifey's for each other fully supporting each other, listening, caring, sharing, showing up and being present.

OK so can you agree to all of this?? If so then by all means dive in slowly, lovingly with great joy because Laura is worth being celebrated.

Now I need to go be with this feeling of giving my Wifey away to a man I do not even know and come to think of it nor does she but....you will soon! :)

Happy Holiday's!

Santa must have been checking his list because he brought you a great, great gift!!!

unwrap slowly....

Travel safely to the west

Julie

Peter's response back:

Hi Love,

My name is Peter and I already feel such a connection and very comfortable in the energy I'm seeing in both of your eyes from Laura's profile pictures of you two. I had to ask Laura if she was for real as I have met a lot of ladies in work-shops, etc., but none that are coming this close to common choices in what we are asking to experience in relationship with our intimate other and how we are seeing all this show up. Anyway, guess I get to see you soon.

Love and Blessings Already in All Ways, Peter

Julie replied to Peter one more time:

Hi Peter

Ok just one more (I promise!) we sisters back each other up and since it is getting closer to the time you meet Laura (of course with no expectations). I also have this to express... just a continuation of what I already shared!!

soooooo....

IT'S NOT WEIRD ANYMORE

Laura is a dear soul sister of mine and if you think she is some ordinary girl she is NOT! She is an extraordinary woman who is a great mystic and has the courage to travel with knives during our most dangerous time on our planet. She does not mess around! She has a sincere heart of gold and cares deeply about uplifting humanity. She is kind and I am sure she is a true and delicious lover and will touch you deeply in your heart and soul to the depths of your manly core of your being. She is to be treasured, adored and even worshipped. For she is a chosen one directly by the sweet divine Goddess herself to be a conduit of the divine feminine energy, penetrating into the hearts, minds and souls of the many on the planet. She is beautiful inside and out. She walks her talk and will only accept a proposal of love that is true and pure. It is her time to love and be loved in a way that is rare now in our world and she will not succumb to anything less than sacred, present, divine companionship. Are you the one to meet her in this way?? If so only bring your authentic male sexual essence of radiance and presence. Seek only to worship and adore the ground that Laura walks upon with great reverence and respect. In this you will awaken in a way you never even dreamed of. If you will only allow the very sacred and feminine essence of my sweet sister friend Laura to penetrate deep into your heart. You will look no further for you will have found a partner in which you will dance your way into your remembering of your enlightenment. She stands before you now with open eyes, with an open authentic heart of gold.

Brother Peter of the path you need only to say yes and smile that you have made this choice!

Sincerely,

and authentically

a sister of the path of the one

Julie

I felt I had a little explaining to do to Peter about carrying knives around. The knives are referring to my ritual tools I use for etheric healing. Emotional Cord Cutting works well with a ritual knife. Energetic cords on the etheric level are formed in any relationship and connect you to another person even when you are apart or no longer together. Once these emotional cords are cut you have renewed energy and can re-establish your present relationships on a new level. The Cord Cutting is beneficial particularly when you are beginning a new romantic relationship and want a clean slate to start the new and leave the old one behind.

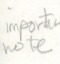

important note

~ 7 ~

My other friend, Cynthia, who checked out Peter's profile, is my feng shui consultant and teacher. We met at a New Age health expo in 1996 where I had a massage booth and she had a feng shui booth. We were immediately drawn to each other and have remained close friends ever since. She is always involved in arranging my new digs wherever I land. This is what she did to my bedroom to energetically prepare and draw Peter to me.

My current living space is a small two-bedroom, one-bath, converted garage healing room with laundry, single-story house. The yard is beautifully landscaped with several large cedar trees that line the entire backyard, with curved walkways, raised garden beds, and an aesthetically pleasing architectural privacy fenced backyard. I believe this is my landlord's artistic expression as well as mine. My expression is on the inside of course. When my roommate moved out to live with her new boyfriend whom I introduced her to a few years ago, the house was very bare. I had very little furniture and kitchen supplies. I went out and bought the basics for the kitchen, a used couch in great shape, and left my new bedroom empty so Cynthia could start from scratch. I waited for her to make time to help me with the decor and placement of things. My bedroom took up most of our time as she turned it into a beautiful, balanced, feminine, masculine lair. I call it the *Queen's Chamber*. The bed is the centerpiece, with a gold comforter with African animals etched in, a body pillow with a leopard print cover as the headboard, two red pillows and a small decorative pillow with red and leopard print covering. Hanging on the wall above the bed is a beautiful batik of a blue lotus flower. The relationship corner to the far right from the entry has a nightstand with a large picture of statues of a divine couple in an erotic embrace sitting on a shelf above it. Cynthia placed a black decorative blanket throw across my bed at an angle that begins at the entrance and is directed toward the erotic couple. She called this "the road to my relationship." She had me place small tiger print rugs on either side of the bed to invite the masculine and feminine in. She also suggested I take away objects that were from past relationships and I wholeheartedly complied. I mounted wall sconces on the two opposing walls on either side of the bed for candles. I bought candle lamps to place on the nightstand on the right and the altar on the left side of the bed. The far left is my wealth corner, where my heirloom table altar sits. I have several sacred objects placed on the altar, the main one being a meditating Jesus as well as things that represent the elements in their specific direction; sand from Egypt in the north for earth, a feather wing in the east for air, an oil candle in the south for fire, and holy water from the Vatican in the west for water. In addition there are a variety of stones that have been given to me for different occasions and last but not least a small saucer plate from Israel designed with a mosaic of the basket of the never ending fishes filled with rice and mala beads holding up a Shiva lingam and a rough ruby to represent the man who is coming; two leopard print vases, one with peacock feathers that sits on the floor next to the altar and another on a shelf above it with silk roses. The opposite wall from the blue lotus batik is a long dresser that has a large, sheer green vase with peacock feathers to the left as you are facing the dresser. A statue of a peacock sits next to it with a decoratively painted heirloom metal box in the middle of the dresser. Above the box hangs an ornate family heirloom picture frame that used to hold an unknown relative. Now it frames an ancient print of a beautiful exotic dancer entertaining a wise, handsome king and queen or lord and lady in their medieval castle and their pet cheetah. A hand-painted gong hangs to the right of the picture. The hall and bedroom doorways are flanked with colorful veils with long fringe, held back with my costume necklaces.

When Cynthia was done placing the last finishing touches I was in awe and felt as if I was waking up inside of a famous painting every morning. I was a little shy about letting any men see my bedroom, particularly my clients, as they must pass by on their way to the bathroom. The *Queen's Chamber* looks like a sensual sex palace and I did not want to appear that way to my male clients, but I proudly showed all my women clients and friends, and they loved it.

The rest of the house is decorated with similar furnishings; a Turkish rug that covers much of the living room wood floor, Buddha heads and full body Buddha statues, ornate metal wall hangings, real and silk plants, and lots of artistic large swatches of material to decorate ceilings and walls, as well as a few mandala wall hangings, the Mayan calendar, and a batique with an elephant head and ohm symbol.

This feng shui job was much faster and easier than the first one Cynthia and I created together. I used to live in an old house with a large unfinished basement, so we turned it into an Egyptian Healing Chamber. We painted the walls with temple-looking stones, Egyptian Deities as big as us, hieroglyphs, and the dark blue Egyptian night sky, complete with scarabs and the multicolored stripes as a decorative border lining the ceiling. To tie it all together I installed a dark purple carpet throughout the whole basement, as there were two bedrooms or healing rooms, an entrance waiting area, and bathroom. It looked magnificent. My landlord called me the sacred tenant. I always knew when I moved out that I would have to paint over the Deities because I had no way of knowing if the next tenants would honor and respect their energy. The day before I moved out, I painted over them and the next day Seattle had one of the largest earthquakes in decades. Some of my friends say I caused it.

Cynthia is definitely one of my Egyptian sisters and I love working with her and creating artistic projects. She can turn any space into a work of art and may save you from remodeling. In addition she has assisted many of her satisfied clients with much better living environments that have helped release stagnant energy within the individual. I greatly value her assistance in opening up my living space to allow Peter to easily join me. Feng shui is a very powerful tool and is listed in the resource section in the back of this book for further reference.

~ 8 ~

Peter and I made plans to meet over the Christmas holidays and decided we would give each other as Christmas presents to one another. I have not been interested in Christmas for years, as the shopping, marketing, guilt-giving event it has appeared to me. This proposal was totally different, exciting, fun, and bold, especially since we had not met physically yet. I had been Match.com dating that fall and with my PGP training, I was very aware of fantasy on the computer. I definitely had a totally different experience with Peter than the other Internet dates. My intuition kept saying yes, yes, yes above my logical thinking mind's protest.

Although I do not celebrate Christmas the traditional way, I wholeheartedly celebrate the Winter Solstice every year with pagan artists in Seattle. We find a warehouse, paint and decorate the place into a medieval palace. This event is a 500-person potluck with incredibly beautiful large art installations that you can dance, walk, sit, lie down, and sleep in. There are many bands, musicians, dancers, skit performers, and rituals to witness. My belly dance teacher, friend, mover and shaker, Delilah, usually has a ritual to put together and perform with her Visionary Dancers, and the Winter Solstice of 2006 was no different. The *Winter Solstice Feast* was on December 22nd, the day before Peter would arrive. Delilah's Visionary Dancers had practiced a beautiful ritual for the feast and I was the centerpiece. I wore a gold lamé goddess gown with a lit candelabra on my head and had 13 dancers wrapped in my colorful red wings. We were given the cue that it was time for our ritual to be executed, by the official artist in charge. I made my way shuffling with 13 Visionary Dancers behind me to the large mandala painted on the floor for our performance. The dancers unfolded from my wings as they danced in circles around me with lighted Christmas balls in their hands. As they passed by they danced in honor of me, as I represented the feminine aspect for the time of year. I held a statuesque pose and made slow mudra movements with my hands and arms as I shook sistrums (Egyptian rattles) at appropriate moments to the rhythms of live music.

I hesitated to invite Peter to this event because I figured I would lose my performance focus and felt it was best for our first meeting to be alone. This way we would have each other's concentrated, focused attention with no interruptions or frustration.

While I lay in my hospital bed I was reminded of a part of my costume that may have been a metaphor about my situation. Delilah and I diligently worked to make a face veil for me to wear that covered my face from just below my eyes to below my chin for the Solstice performance. The reasoning at the time was in case the candelabra became heavy from wearing it for a long time no one could see any strain on my face. I believe this was a loving sendoff for my new facial metamorphosis. Interesting to think about as my experience with Delilah exposes many metaphors and archetypes as she creates performance pieces that play out in our lives. My relationship/friendship with her has been quite magickal.

~ 9 ~

Delilah and I met back in 1990 during my first marriage, to Gary, at my sister-

IT'S NOT WEIRD ANYMORE

in-law Sarah's house. Sarah's husband, George, was the drummer in a rock and roll band called Junior Cadillac, a 24-year-old northwest band in 1990. Junior Cadillac was in Russia having a rock and roll exchange in Tashkent. They were scheduled to air on the radio, and Sarah, Gary, and my in-laws, George and Jane, met at Sarah's to listen together and my mom, Liz, happened to be with us as well. When Gary, Liz, and I arrived we were introduced to Delilah and her two small precocious children, Laura Rose and Victoria. Delilah's husband, Steve, was the keyboard player and the newest member of the band as he had been with them for ten years at that time. Mom and I were instantly attracted to Delilah and stayed in close, intense, intimate conversation the whole visit. It was almost as if no one else was present, while Delilah seemed to be helping Mom and me remember something about our feminine power and roots. The three of us appeared to be lost in one another's essence as we re-remembered ourselves and our distant past lives together. That was my interpretation of the feeling in that moment.

My connection with Delilah was to become of enormous importance as my marriage to Gary came to an end. My first marriage appeared to be all about making money and spending it on construction projects. I was a blue-collar worker splicing high-voltage cable for Seattle City Light and extremely masculine. I had worked blue-collar jobs at that point for 20 years. I began commercial fishing in Alaska in my late teens, early twenties as a deckhand, moved on to deckhand on a mini cruise ship, then able-bodied seaman (woman) on seagoing tugboats to Alaska. When Gary and I met he was working on oilrigs in the North Sea out of Scotland as a life support technician for the deep-sea oil divers.

We built a beautiful 32-foot modified Herreshoff sailboat with a mahogany cabin, teak deck, and yellow cedar interior that we lived on in cramped style for four years in Winslow on Bainbridge Island, Washington. We decided we would rather be together than work so far apart, so we both received employment with Seattle City Light. He became a lineman and I became an underground cable-splicer. Before we sold our sailboat we bought a really rotten house in a fancy Seattle neighborhood, Magnolia, to rebuild despite my protest at another construction project. The sailboat was never in my opinion used for the fun it was designed for, considering the extent of all the laborious construction effort.

Looking back, I had a few otherworldly experiences while living with Gary and working at the power company. Before Gary and I began deconstructing and remodeling our house we would observe the landscaping and discuss our vision for the new yard. One day we were standing on our dilapidated back deck overlooking our small backyard and observed a perfectly round indentation that filled the circumference of the grass, which was not there when we moved in. This became a ritual for a few years; we would stand looking down at the indentation and ask the same question over and over again.

"What could that be from?"

Around the same timeframe I had a consistent experience while building transformers alone in the back of the power company work truck. Several times I could feel and hear people walk right up behind me and I thought they were my coworkers. I would turn around to communicate and no one would appear to be there. This happened so many times I started talking to them and expressed my wish to physically see them. There were other times at home and picnics where I could feel strong vortexes surround me. My intuition and logic told me these were my space brothers and sisters raising my frequency and somehow my electrical skills were linked.

A very dear psychic friend told me that the indentation in my yard was from a scout observer ship that was checking me out, because I appeared to be more open-minded to work with. She also said my own energy frequency worked with the power lines to create the electrical energy in a way that the ETs could use for their ships. I have no idea how to scientifically or logically explain this. I believe someday soon all will be revealed and I assume it won't be weird anymore.

Okay, back to the more earthly account.

Despite how busy I was working overtime and coming home to work on our construction projects, I kept Delilah on my mind. She and I would call each other once a year and talk for a few hours. She would ask when was I going to start belly dancing with her? I would answer with something like, after I finish building the workshop garage or some other project I didn't really want to do. Delilah was unaware that she was my lifeline, slowly pulling me into myself. I was pretty depressed and miserable in those days, forcing myself to build Gary's projects. I began to become aware of just how much I repressed my happiness to fit with what I believed was Gary and his family's image of me. I felt like a fraud to myself and had other things I would rather be spending my time cultivating. Finally in the spring of 1993 I moved out, because it was the only way I could see an end to these projects and the beginning of a happier life.

Even though I sound miserable in my marriage to Gary, it was not always like that. Gary and I had a passionate, magickal beginning and recognized each other from past lives. In my opinion life is all about choice and what we choose to experience with our self and others. There is no one to blame for our chosen experiences with each other. I learned a lot about myself in my 12-year relationship with Gary and am enormously grateful for the opportunity to do so. The greatest gift he gave me was helping me work through my sexual hang-up. I primarily hated sex and avoided it at all cost. Spontaneously one night Gary invited me to sexually mount him and tell him how much I hated sex while softly beating on him. I was completely cleared of hating sex after that and was saddened that it was toward the end of our relationship. I believe all our relationships are blessings on our path to know thyself and the hardest personal growth workshop on earth.

I moved in with a close friend, Carol, from the power company on Queen Anne Hill in Seattle and began going to massage school at night while I spliced cable during the day. I remember feeling extremely unbalanced in my body as my masculine side dominated. The right side of the body is the masculine and the left side is the feminine and I literally dragged the left side of my body around with my right. Soon after massage school I ventured out dancing to large community dances where I ran into Delilah. I had to re-introduce myself to her because our relationship was over the phone and we had only physically seen each other once. Massage and belly dancing helped open up my feminine side immensely and my body began to come into balance. I remembered how much I loved to dance and that it was a large part of my life before my marriage.

The summer of 1993 my father was diagnosed with another malignant tumor on his neck and I took time off from work from the power company to care for him. This was another major event during the time of my marriage separation and foremost turning point in my life.

After 12 years of battling cancer my dad was experiencing his last tumor. I decided to help him heal through natural medicine and learn about natural healing methods for myself. I had just finished massage school and practiced massage on the side while splicing high-voltage cable for the power company during the day. We found a naturopath who gave oxygen therapy treatments to boost Dad's immune system. Receiving oxygen therapy five days a week for five weeks raised his immune system from 25% up to 95%. In addition Dad's diet changed to more raw, organic, whole foods, and receiving massages from me was the best he felt. A major problem we were up against was a recent tumor removal surgery where his shoulder met his neck, there were some cut nerves that were painfully growing back together and Dad was put on morphine to ease the pain. This brought his immune system down again and he became weaker. I learned then that I wanted to know why there was so much illness in this country.

This is going to sound really strange but I believe after years of studying natural healing and the cancer-causing chemicals in personal care products that my Dad's illness was caused by a famous mouthwash. First he had two-thirds of his tongue cut out, and the rest of the tumors were all around his throat. He was not a smoker and didn't drink to speak of. Statistics show that there are 36,000 cases of mouth cancer a year from our poison oral hygiene personal care products and 500 deaths a year from the alcohol ingestion.

During the time I took care of my dad I began to lose interest in my day job and gathered the courage to quit the power company and open a full-time private practice as a massage therapist. Life-threatening illnesses usually help us look at what is really important, while all the petty drama seems to melt away. My soon-to-be ex-husband, Gary, and I were going in two totally different directions and thank God we decided to get real about it.

By winter of 1994 Gary and I peacefully divorced with no kids and have remained distant friends. By spring I found my own large rental home in Ballard and was very satisfied that it had finished sheetrock and no construction going on. I had enough of feeling enslaved to property ownership and small, cramped spaces.

That same spring my dad quietly passed away knowing he was very much loved by all the care my mom and I provided. I was grateful for the time I spent reading him stories he would never have read on his own; *Women Who Run with Wolves, Angel Stories,* and *Message from Down Under.* I felt very close and complete with my dad.

After losing both men, quitting my job, moving, and starting my own business, it took some time to reorient myself to my new life. I felt a newfound sense of freedom and at the same time felt like an adult virgin having to re-learn to be single again in an older version of myself, 38 years old to be exact. Dating had changed—either that or I had changed, probably a bit of both. Thank the Goddess for girlfriends; they are the ones who helped me get back in step with myself and answered all my crazy, naive questions. My two most important subjects, spirituality and dancing, were missing in my marriage to Gary, so I made them a priority. I may have gone a little overboard with new potential dates when I introduced myself and launched into the weirdest out there spiritual stuff I could think of. My attitude was I did not want to waste my time with men who could not converse with me about spiritual matters. I am sure I scared a few away, which was the point. There was one man who stayed right with me in the conversation and even added his spiritual viewpoint—now that really turned me on.

I began a new relationship with a beautiful Senegalese Greo (storyteller) Shaman percussionist, Pappys (pronounced Popeace). He was in the process of a divorce and I had just received one. We just wanted to date for a long, long time and have fun playing music and dancing, and we did for seven years. My most fond memories are of Pappys playing in a Reggae band and me trance dancing to his songs. He was instrumental in nurturing my feminine and creative side. He had seven wonderful kids from two different marriages and was a good co-parent.

Pappys and Peter have almost the exact same handwriting and both write poetry. I mentioned this to a psychic friend and she said,

"That's because they are related."

I hypothesize that this is more Egyptian soul connections and not weird at all.

Belly dancing, art, travel, my massage practice, and health became my focus. Delilah and I became closer as I studied with her. I accompanied her to belly dance festivals to help with her belly dance sales booth while dancers performed all day long. She sold her famous Hawaiian Belly Dance Retreat spots, her belly dance instruction videos, and her husband Steve's Middle-Eastern music. It wasn't until I experienced these festivals that I noticed the cat-fighting between belly dance philosophies. My introduction to belly dancing through Delilah was a sisterhood that embodied the Goddess, a beautiful, nonverbal prayer. In my early days of learning the dance and attending these festivals there was a faction of Christian dancers who wanted nothing to do with the Goddess and were very angry with Delilah. She was venomously ridiculed for this for years and she was one of the main dancers who brought the Goddess back into the dance. Now its mainstream thought, thank Goddess.

Delilah and Steve Flynn (her talented musician husband at the time) created these wonderful yearly winter Belly Dance Retreats in Hawaii beginning in 1993, which are still being created and offered at the time of this writing. I could not wait to attend and was able to participate in my first one in 1995 where I met Wifey. We took belly dancing from Delilah and other guest teachers as well as drumming lessons and took trips dancing in nature and into the ocean. There was a boating day with all the dancers dancing onboard and snorkeling in costume where the fish approached and nibbled on shells that hung from our mermaid swimming attire. On this particular day humpback whales swam right up to the boat, so close we could pet them. The captain said he had been sailing out here for years and had never experienced this before. He seemed to sense our group possessed a magickal quality and had made an extra effort to be the belly dancer retreat captain. There was a dancing-into-the-sea costume contest as well as performance evenings with themes, and all of the excursions and events were to fabulous live music.

Delilah and I have a very strong Egyptian connection and decided to take a trip together. In addition to being a world-famous belly dancer she is also a whirling dervish, the Sufi spiritual mystics who wear large round white skirts and long white top hats as they spin and spin and spin a cosmic orbit dance. Delilah's Turkish Sheik Jaleluddin Loras of the Mevlevi Order of America was leading a group of American Sufi whirling dervishes to Turkey in November of 1997 to Konya where Rumi's tomb is enshrined. Women are not allowed to spin/turn in Turkey, so Jaleluddin decided to take American women dervishes to perform the task. The goal was to receive permission to perform a dervish celestial dance in Rumi's tomb to live music. Rumi was a famous 13th-century Persian poet who inspired the Sufi movement. We were not allowed to discuss with the Turks what we were there to do. Cool! I loved the idea of being on a secret mission in a foreign land. Delilah and I determined that we would begin our trip with the dervishes for ten days and then take off on our own to Egypt for three and a half weeks. Our Turkish tour consisted of half women and half men, about 25 people in all. This expedition deserves its own chapter as it is quite a lengthy adventure and a very significant part of my life and reinforces the Egyptian links that continue to appear throughout the course of my life.

~ 10 ~

The first three days of our journey were open and free-flowing as we landed in Cappadocia, a hobbit-looking landscape with caves and long, tall, soft rock formations that looked a lot like penises including the head.

Upon our first day of exploration we met Memet in his carpet shop and he became extremely curious to know who we were. He looked at the way we were dressed, I guess kind of hippie dervish like. He asked in his polished English,

"Where is your spaceship and what planet are you from? You don't look like regular tourists."

Delilah and I gave each other a question mark look and then Delilah turned and locked eyes with Memet in a silent, you could hear a pin drop pause. Is it safe to answer truthfully? We wondered. Anyone who would ask that kind of question deserves the truth, Delilah and I psychically agreed. With their eyes still locked and Delilah's right eyebrow raised she said,

"You know, we're dervishes."

Delilah and I wondered what kind of reaction we would get as she spilled the beans. Memet became completely intrigued, honored, and wanted to know everything and asked if he could be our escort that night.

After a day of discovery Delilah and I dressed up for a night on the town to meet our two carpet guys, Memet and Memet, two cousins we had agreed could show us around. They picked us up at our hotel and took us disco cave dancing. We had a very insightful, stimulating conversation between dances and planned to meet again the next night for a belly dance show. We thanked Memet and Memet for the subsequent invitation and informed them we were belly dancers. They looked puzzled and said,

"Dervishes can't be belly dancers too."

This was so intriguing and foreign to them; we felt like we were changing their reality before their very eyes, and they wanted more. I love this about traveling the most, meeting people from different cultures and backgrounds and exchanging thoughts and ideas that change and open your mind to other thoughts and ideas. For me traveling is one of my highest forms of education. When I connect with the people of the area I feel as though I have made an intimate, authentic union with the country.

On our second-day excursion before our second night out with Memet and Memet, Delilah and I ventured up an elevated area in Cappadocia for the view. We looked down and around at the different rock formations with ancient temples carved inside the soft basalt hills; it was an amazing sight. Two thousand years ago Christians lived inside the carved-out hills and when an invading army encroached upon them, they covered over the main entryway with a large round boulder. The invaders never knew there were 10,000 people living inside the hills and the intruders would peacefully move on past.

While we enjoyed our surroundings, Delilah recognized a Hawaiian Belly Dance Retreat dancer, Mishal, and her artistic musician husband, Goro. Delilah and Mishal were pleasantly surprised and ran to greet each other. Delilah was reminded that Mishal sent her a letter just before we left Seattle that said she was traveling to Turkey. Delilah had a premonition that she would meet Mishal somewhere along our journey—interesting how it was only our second day in Turkey. Mishal mentioned she and Goro were going to a belly dance show that same night, and of course it happened to be the same one we were attending with our Memets.

Memet and Memet, our 25-year-old dates, picked up their 42- and 43-year-old dates at the hotel again and brought us straight to the dinner and show. It was a large tourist attraction as there were maybe 150 people seated in long family-style picnic/conference tables circling the room. The center of the room was reserved for the performers. We sat with Mishal, Goro, and many others, eating delicious Mediterranean food while we waited for the show to start.

Finally a petite, young, very skilled belly dancer appeared as she hypnotized us with her undulating serpentine moves. Delilah and I talked with her while she visited our table and asked where she learned to dance so beautifully and she said her aunt had initiated her into the dance.

The next performer was a long, thin, wispy guy who moved more like a real snake than any performer I have seen before. He kept us entertained and laughing with drunken members from the audience being brought into the performance to badly mimic belly dancing. Then he asked Delilah, Mishal, and another dancer to join him, not knowing they were professional dancers while they outperformed him.

It was a fun, touristy night and Delilah and I knew it would be our last since we would be headed to the religious city of Konya to behave like quiet, honorable women in the morning. When we arrived back at our hotel we were greeted by some seriously concerned Sufis who assumed we were troublemakers because we were not behaving like virtuous women by staying out late dancing and partying. They were alarmed that Delilah and I would continue going out at night, having fun with strange men, and jeopardizing our chances of turning in Rumi's Tomb. We assured our fellow dervishes we knew this was our last night out in this manor and would behave like reverent, unassuming, modest women from this point on.

The women in our group were asked to cover our bodies from head, neck, and down to our toes, just like the strict religious region of Konya that we were traveling to. This would help our group receive permission to spin in Rumi's Tomb. It was extremely important that we did not draw attention to ourselves, anything that would give the officials a reason to keep our group from our spiritual ritual performance in the tomb.

We arrived at our hotel, which was situated across the street from the Turkish Museum that housed Rumi. The museum was designed with beautiful Arabic architecture as Rumi lay inside a tall, magnificent, turquoise conical turret. Our group of half men and covered-up American women descended upon the museum as curious tourists. We were quite an anomaly to the regular tourists and the locals. The regular tourists thought we were authentic, traditional religious Muslim Turks and took their touristy pictures of us for their photo travel albums. The locals stared at us with curiosity as it was obvious to them we were not authentic. Delilah was completely covered in black and could feel a modernly dressed Turkish woman glaring at her. Delilah imagined her thought to be, *What are you doing? I worked hard to overcome and remove myself from that repressive religious tradition.*

We stood in front of Rumi's burial tomb, perched high above us and covered in intricate gold cloth; the decorative tomb appeared to climb high up into the tall conical cone it rested in. The conical walls were filled with sacred Arabic calligraphy and ascended up into what seemed like infinity. The energy that surrounded the tomb was powerfully positive and many of us were moved to tears. I believe this energy was a result of all the positive prayers from the many visitors and created a vortex of uplifting energy.

Back in the privacy of our hotel room, we stripped down, seeking relief from the 100-degree heat, and waited in obscurity until we were granted permission to whirl as a dervish in the poet's tomb.

Delilah and I ventured out the next day sightseeing and shopping in our completely covered look, complete with a video camera. We strolled along the open market shops as I filmed Delilah leading the tour with her animated commentary. We accepted an invitation into a carpet shop where we would have tea and be able to film. Our Turkish male host commented that we looked like Turkish spies with our bodies covered from head to toe and carrying a video camera. Video cameras in 1997 were still quite large, cumbersome, and very visible, not like the matchbox size made today.

Delilah filmed my interview with our host as I asked him what he thought about women being totally covered in the 100-degree heat. He said I looked lovely in my headscarf, long sleeves, and long skirt. He did not seem to have a clue about any discomfort women may have. I suppose the women who have accepted dressing this way day in and day out may not think about it either.

Delilah and I returned to the other shops and were met with such curiosity about why we were dressed like local women, but obviously not able to pull it off. We stuck to our agreement and did not divulge our group's secret mission. Someone asked me why I was wearing a headscarf if I was not a Turkish Muslim woman and I replied,

"I had cancer."

Finally after three days of waiting to receive permission, we got it! The dervishes ironed their four-yard white circle skirts and tunic tops. I slipped into my evergreen East Indian spiritual best Turkish outfit and walked across the street to the museum with our entourage. The local musicians followed and began setting up their instruments in the stage cubby. The dervishes lined up to receive Sheik Jaleluddin's position instructions and formed a celestial circle in the main large round room as they waited for the musicians to finish setting up. I set up the video camera to document the event and felt as if I was filming for Public Television's *The American Experience*.

The live Turkish music began as the dervish planets slowly began to whirl and take their place in the celestial dance. It was magnificent and too bad that the locals could not witness it. I saw one young Turkish woman, who was the daughter of an official, watching in wonderment while my camera caught her looking directly into the lens. Our group was informed that the local dervishes had never been allowed to spin in the museum at the foot of Rumi's Tomb. I felt privileged to witness and take part in this historic, once-in-a-lifetime event and hopefully anchor the sacred feminine energy in this place. The depth of emotion was truly indescribable.

IT'S NOT WEIRD ANYMORE

Okay, mission accomplished! The next leg of our journey we toured the rest of Turkey and circle-danced our way around the country. The main historic stop was to Ephesus on the coast, part of the Greek ruins and the supposed resting place of Mother Mary. Delilah and I enjoyed swimming in a tremendously large natural hot springs filled with Roman ruins of broken columns just outside of Ephesus. Travel can be extraordinarily surreal when the ancient and the modern meet. I feel like my ancient past life memory becomes stimulated and triggered in places of antiquity.

I became the healer in the back of our tour bus with my new skills using essential oils and massage experience. Our group of Sufis came to me for aches, pains, depression, constipation, counseling, comfort, and love. The most eye-opening observation being on the back of the bus provided was watching the bus attendant collect all our garbage, bring it to the back door, and throw it out of the moving bus. I, along with other observers, were appalled by this.

Our dervish caravan traveled north on the east coast of Turkey, stopping in more obscure places to whirl in the circle dance while Delilah and I contemplated the next leg of our journey to Egypt on our own. Our bus driver hurried to a small town airport to drop us off for our flight to Istanbul. The driver came around a tight corner entrance to a very narrow average street, became stuck, and blocked traffic. The Turks got out of their cars and proceeded to yell at the bus driver while a policeman tried helping by directing the bus in a difficult, time-consuming situation. Delilah and I made the observation that this would take longer than we had time to wait for our flight. We quickly said our tearful good-byes to Jaleluddin and our Sufi sisters and brothers, and hailed a cab.

Once in the small airport, we realized that there was no signage in English and we could not communicate with the airport personnel. Boy! Did we feel lost and helpless. The personnel motioned us to a small office to sit and wait. In the meantime Delilah and I calmed ourselves down with a prayer for an angel's guidance. Soon a handsome young Turkish man in an airline pilot uniform entered the office and said,

"I will help you."

We smiled at him with a long exhale of relief, thanked him, and knew he was the angel we requested. He was cute too!

The young, handsome pilot was not to fly the plane, but was a passenger who happened to be going the same direction we were. He accompanied us with his friendly, angelic, polite presence, answering our questions about himself. He worked as a pilot on a private jet for a wealthy family business, had flown all over the world and told us the Istanbul airport was the worst airport on the planet. His guidance did not stop once we landed; he proceeded to escort us all the way through the extremely confusing airport to our connecting flight to Cairo. We graciously thanked him for being our angel guide and pleased to have an escort after our traumatic first impression at the beginning of our trip in this same airport. I broke down crying after personnel after personnel gave us the wrong directions to our flight gate, or so I perceived it that way. Since then the Istanbul airport has been completely remodeled and is one of the best airports in the world today.

Delilah and I landed at night in Cairo while I had nausea and diarrhea to contend with. Thank Goddess we knew where we were sleeping and scheduled some down time. We were booked at the three-star Victoria Hotel with Victorian design and character, and I spent the next day in bed recovering from my illness.

Delilah planned our next adventure in Cairo, since the Egyptian part of our trip was spontaneous except where we slept at night. In Egypt all costs are always negotiable, so we paid for our hotel rooms in advance through Queens Tours in order to have control over how much money we spent. The hotel destinations ranged from Cairo, Luxor, Aswan, and all the way up the Nile to Abu Simbel as well as a Nile cruise. We were the only queens on the tour.

After a day of rest at the hotel and me feeling much better, we ventured out on a walk to find the Queens Tours office and check in. Cairo is very smoggy, the outside of the buildings look atrociously dirty, and many buildings look dilapidated and abandoned. We followed our directions and walked past the building chaos and found the address we were looking for. We found a set of stairs to climb to the sixth floor and became disenchanted when each floor we passed was destroyed and torn apart with piles of broken glass. We began to think we had been ripped off and there was no such thing as the Queens Tours, but something prompted us to keep going and we continued to climb the stairs. When we arrived on the sixth floor, we entered a palatial space with red carpet and well-dressed Queens Tour greeters. This seemed so crazy to us.

We asked about the other floors and were told that the downtown Cairo buildings were never allowed to raise their rent on their current tenants by a law that was passed twenty years before. Tenants did not move out and the building owners could not afford to keep them fixed up so they let them deteriorate. In addition when a building is finished the owner must begin paying property taxes, so the structures are never completed. Sounds like everyone lost. So when a company wants to have a downtown office they are obliged to fix it up themselves.

This was the beginning of our learning curve into the Egyptian system. Pay no attention to streetlights and pedestrian crosswalks because they will not keep you from being injured or killed. Look in every direction and take your chances crossing the street because drivers pay no attention to lane markers; they just fill in empty spaces. Egyptian police do not hand out traffic tickets as our beautiful youthful Queens Tour office guide pointed out. She said she was side swiped and her side-view mirror broken off; she took down the license plate and found a policeman to report it to. When she finished explaining what happened he said,

"Ask Allah to avenge him."

The men at Queens Tours seemed a little puzzled by two women traveling alone and kept a close eye on our travel plans. We received an overview of what excursions were available in the different cities and directions to the pyramids at the Giza Plateau for the afternoon, then said our farewells and were off.

IT'S NOT WEIRD ANYMORE

We caught a cab and asked where we could rent camels and ride to the pyramids. The cabdriver dropped us off where camels and horses were hanging around in front of a small shop. We negotiated with the shopkeeper and came to an agreed upon roundtrip price. Our main tour guide and two young boys came with the package and led us away from their shop and toward the grand, magnificent, ancient structures that take you back to a long ago golden age. We actually rented a horse and camel, so Delilah and I traded places every so often. When we came upon the Sphinx I was reminded that I could imagine what the nose actually looked like. Pappys, my boyfriend at the time, appeared to have the rest of the facial features depicted by the Sphinx, so I imagined the face intact with Pappys' nose.

Delilah and I plodded along, led by our young camel and horse escorts, while the guide joked and teased us with probing questions in an attempt to find out a little about who we were. He seemed particularly interested that Delilah was a professional belly dancer and invited us to a wedding that was scheduled in three days. He said a belly dancer was performing at the wedding and suggested Delilah would be better and should come. We were very tempted to attend as guests but were scheduled to be in Luxor with paid for Hilton reservations, so we chose to keep to our specific city plans.

Our whirling dervish comrades were scheduled to spin at a big event in Istanbul this same day and agreed to psychically connect with us. How appropriate that we would be touring the great pyramids to hook up with them. We parked our camel and horse below the entrance and climbed the stone pathway and waited at the entrance for a number of tourists to exit before we could enter. Our wait was not boring as we were entertained by young women belly dancing to live drums below in the desert sand. Delilah and I danced with them and waved to one another in recognition. Soon we walked through the entryway and stood still to feel the energy while the guard asked Delilah if she would like to pray. I thought, *How could he know that, how strange.* Delilah let me know that she was standing in front of me with her arms crossed, her hands holding onto her shoulders, one of the prayer stances for dervishes. The guard kind of adopted us and began to give us a private tour.

Delilah brought about fifty pictures of herself dressed as Hathor in front of an Egyptian backdrop at an Isis temple in California to give away to the guards and whoever seemed appropriate.

Hathor is the patron of the sky, the sun, the queen, music, dance, and the arts. She appears as a cow bearing the sun disk between her horns, or a woman in queenly raiment wearing the sun disk and horns on her head. Many followers of Hathor were artisans, musicians, and dancers who turned their talents into creating rituals that were beautiful works of art. Music and dance were part of the worship of Hathor like no other deity in Egypt. Delilah definitely depicts these traits; therefore she is the perfect embodiment of Hathor since knowing her personally and for the magickal journey that lay ahead.

LAURA LEGERE

Our new guide led us to a closed-off Queens Chamber entrance and said he was sorry it was locked for restoration, but we could stand and pray. Delilah and I placed our hands on the outside stonewalls and silently chanted a Sufi chant. I cannot remember the words but the intention and energy felt powerful in our quiet, meditative state. The guard stayed close by, ready to guide us to the Kings Chamber. We were directed up a wooden walkway and soon entered a large room with a high ceiling and could see the apex of the great pyramid as we slowly strolled around the room. We stood still in the center of the acoustically accurate chamber and began toning to connect with our dervish comrades while loads of tourists whizzed by with their curious stares. The tones reverberated around us as we imagined our sound reaching out through the pyramid walls, over the land, across the water, and connecting to our whirling friends.

We then followed our guide to the stone sarcophagus in the far corner of the chamber and Delilah climbed in and lay down to meditate for 60 seconds. After Delilah removed herself I was motioned to enter the stone coffin, lie down, and meditate. The half wall structure around the sarcophagus was somewhat deeper than I anticipated and our guide was standing a little too close for my smooth leg swing to climb over the wall and into the tomb. As I swung my leg over the edge, my foot kicked our gracious host right in the balls. He bent over in pain while I profusely apologized and wondered how I could be calm and meditate after such a dramatic entrance. I lay down on the cold stone and tried to preoccupy my mind with a silent chant anyway. After about a minute I was prodded by Delilah to stand up and exit the sarcophagus. Our guide seemed to have recovered from my accidental attack on his private parts and escorted us toward the entry door. Delilah attempted to give him one of her Hathor pictures, but he waved her off thinking it was money and indicated we were not finished with our private showing.

He guided us back down the wooden walkway, pointed to a locked steel gate, and asked if we wanted to investigate. He apologized for not having a key and whispered for us to climb over while he looked around to make sure no one was near and motioned us to climb fast. In our long summer dresses Delilah and I, as modestly as possible, jumped over the tall steel gate and wondered where we were going. Our guide moved in front and led our way down a three-foot-high narrow tunnel. I was forced to carry my backpack on my stomach because I was too tall for the low ceiling. Delilah, our guide, and I crawled on all fours down the small space. We traveled for what felt like a mile because it took about a half hour to reach the bottom to a large rough-looking open room. There only appeared to be natural rough rock formations, no hieroglyphs, sarcophagus, or statues. The Great Cheops pyramid has no hieroglyphs anywhere as far as has been discovered or disclosed to the public. The only formation that looked manmade was a small kind of shallow, dry canal in the center of the room among the rough rock formations. Our guide clasped our hands and moved us in the center to tone while the three of us huddled arm to shoulder in a circle. He acted as if he had done this several times before and knew just what spiritual foreigners wanted to experience. Delilah and I

IT'S NOT WEIRD ANYMORE

sat down on a small rock platform in the narrow canal facing each other and sang the Sufi chant while looking deep into each other's eyes and cried. Our emotions were very influenced by the energy we tapped into. Later we discovered that this was the dead center bottom of the pyramid. I read that the reason the tunnel to the bottom center was closed was because several people actually died from mysterious circumstances. A whole group of people died in the bottom chamber from strange fumes that were never understood or found. Some people died from snake and spider bites that are not native and never found in the tunnel or the country for that matter. My resource suggested that the tunnel and its chamber is a fourth dimensional vortex and people can manifest their fears quite literally.

Soon it was time to head out and up the long claustrophobic tunnel back to the real world. We decided to give our host a $30 tip in American money before the climb back up, so I handed him $10 and Delilah gave him $20. He seemed unsatisfied and communicated that he wanted another $10 from me. We were totally surprised at his reaction, gave him the extra $10, and began to think we had an unauthentic experience with him. Before this exchange it felt like an otherworldly encounter, a real mysterious adventure. We crawled the long way up the tunnel to the locked gate, climbed back over to a curious group of tourists watching and wondering where we had come from. A couple of young men came over and asked what I had seen; keeping with my sworn-to-secrecy vow to our guide, I pretended I could not speak English. Even if I spoke I could not begin to explain what I had experienced in that moment anyway. Our guide spoke to us in his very broken English and handed back my $10 bill. He asked if we wanted to come back the next day and said not to tell anyone, otherwise his job would be kyboshed. When we received the $10 bill back we felt as if our guide may have had some sort of emotional experience, which felt better to us. On the other hand it may have been his way of luring us back the next day for another ride. We liked the option of returning the next day, but had no idea if we would. What a profound and amazing first day of travel in Egypt. I don't always have words to describe how these experiences affect me, but it's as if I am going back in time, tracing my footsteps, and something inside of me is activated for future use. It's hard to know for sure, but trusting my intuition about these things feels right.

We exited the pyramid and found our other guide patiently waiting for our return. He asked if we had made our phone call, meaning did we connect with our dervish friends in Turkey; at least we thought that's what he meant. I believe we may have been inside longer than most. Anyway, we mounted our horse and camel, proceeded down the plateau into downtown Khufu and back to our guide's small shop. When it was time for us to pay the bill it became apparent that we were going to be charged a different price than what was negotiated before our little excursion. Of course it wasn't less expensive; welcome to Egypt, this is the way it is.

Our cabdriver stood close by patiently waiting to safely return us to Cairo. He was an enjoyable, friendly fellow and had agreed to be our driver for the day at a reasonable price. He dropped us at our hotel and arranged to be our guide around the city the next day as well.

Delilah and I had fun shopping for belly dance costumes directly from the famous seamstresses who are well known in the United States. We welcomed our driver to join us in our shopping excursion and he seemed to be entertained and enjoying himself as much we were. He took us to a very large store that had three floors of belly dance costumes and accessories; we were astounded and hypnotized, as we had never seen so many sparkly garments in one place. Delilah tried on outfit after outfit; we were in there forever.

Delilah would tell the driver what she was looking for and he knew where to take us every time. We visited the Cairo Museum on this day; saw King Tut's tomb and the many mysterious ancient artifacts that permeate the building. I wondered what was in the basement; now that would be worth exploring; I would love to do that, but of course it was off limits.

We arrived back in our hotel room to pack and prepare for our departure flight in the morning to Luxor. We were greeted at the airport by our Queens Tours guides to make sure we safely boarded our plane. They seemed nervous about two women traveling alone and appeared a bit overprotective to us.

We arrived at the Luxor Hilton, unpacked, and ventured out to explore the area. The entrance to the hotel had a charming Middle Eastern band playing that consisted of two old men, one blind on the *doumbek* drums, and a young man playing a primitive stringed instrument called a *rebabba*. Delilah began to belly dance to their familiar rhythms and as usual developed quite a few local fans. The young rebabba musician communicated in very broken English that he would like us to meet his family. We accepted along with our nonexistent Arabic communication skills. He hailed a cab and we all piled in and were driven to an old village with mud walls and straw roofs not too far from the Hilton, although Delilah and I had no idea where we were. Our young musician friend led us to a house where a young woman invited us in and we were guided to a small room. There was a wide language barrier so we used sign language to compensate as best we could. The small room consisted of a bed, a window, a nightstand, and a well-worn ghetto blaster with paint spatterings all over it. Our new friend motioned for us to sit on his bed while he put in a tape and began to belly dance for us. We were in total amazement with our mouths dropped open as he entertained us with his confident skills and talent as a belly dancer. We asked how he learned and he said by watching videos.

Next he showed the way on foot down the narrow, unpaved streets through the village to his family's residence. We were cheerfully greeted by his sisters, brother, mother, and young children—not sure whose children they were. Our gracious host was anxious to show us something as he stood on the stone couch and excitedly plucked the only picture frame in the room from a live electrical wire hook that sparked while he pulled the picture from the wall. He handed it to Delilah and me to read and to our surprise it was a music award from Washington,

IT'S NOT WEIRD ANYMORE

DC and only a month old. Our host was part of a cultural music event in North America last month, how cool! We congratulated him with recognition, honor, and excitement.

We sat in a half circle in the main living-gathering room on pillows that lay on top of a mud bench that matched the rough adobe walls. Our host's brother could speak English a little better and helped us communicate. A group of neighbors tried to enter the home with baskets of trinkets for us to buy and were waved off by our new friend's mother. This indicated to Delilah and I that we were not regular tourists and this was a very special visit.

Soon we danced for the small family audience as they clapped, ziggurated, and joined in the dance. Music and dance are always universal languages, and I look forward to the day when this is how we interact with all cultures, and war, bigotry, and ignorance have been long forgotten.

Delilah admired the caftan the mother wore and took her up on her offer to try it on and purchase the beautiful navy blue and white-embroidered garment. She looked elegant in it with her long, dark curly hair and deep-sea blue eyes.

Delilah and I were beginning to feel like a captive audience after a while and did not know where we were or what time it was and felt it was time to leave. We indicated that we would like to get back to our hotel and were directed outside to two horses waiting for us to climb onto. I started to protest a little under my breath, something about riding a camel the day before and being sore. Delilah looked down at me from her horse and in her commanding voice said,

"Don't make a scene and get on."

Two young Egyptian men escorted our horses as we sauntered our way through the unpaved streets and adobe straw-roofed village. Young children would run after our horses chanting hello, hello, hello and we would say hello back as they giggled. Delilah and I would say the Arabic greeting, *Salaam Alaikum* (peace be to you), as we passed by the villagers on the road. I felt as if we were in biblical times and imagined this society to be that far left in time.

We arrived in an open area away from buildings where people gathered to socialize and kids played. All of a sudden Delilah and I felt small pebbles being thrown at us and shouts of,

"Sharmoota."

Delilah said,

"I know what that means, it means whore in Arabic."

Our horses began to get spooked and we became nervous and uncomfortable. We both told our guides in a stern, firm voice that we were dismounting now! We took our horses reins and led them behind our young escorts through the dirt street a short distance and safely away from the open social area as the tense episode was over in a flash. We wondered where we were going and how much further. Delilah looked over at me, with her head scarf and long dress, holding onto the reins of her horse, walking through a mud hut village, and asked me in her strained voice,

LAURA LEGERE

"Where's the Hilton?"

Her question caught me by surprise in that particular moment and I began to laugh at the extreme appearance of it all. Her question was answered soon after it was asked because the Hilton was surprisingly around the next corner.

Back in our hotel room we took a nap and freshened up for the evening show downstairs. Our new friend belly dancing with his band was the night's entertainment. Delilah took him up on his invitation to partner belly dance, so he placed a broom handle belly to belly. They danced in synchronistic union with their undulating, artistic movements, appearing unconcerned with the broom handle that separated them. Soon our friend gave Delilah the spotlight and let her dance solo as she mesmerized the crowd with her hypnotic performance. The hotel staff was so impressed that Delilah was handed a dance contract at our dinner table to sign right then and there. It was a nice gesture, but Delilah had two young teenagers and a husband at home waiting for her return.

The Hilton Hotel lobby was filled with all kinds of expeditions to pick from, so Delilah and I made fast friends with one of the travel coordinators, Sammy, to help us decide what to do. Karnac and Luxor temples were close by, the Valley of the Kings and Queens was across the Nile, Dendera was a long one-and-a-half-hour cab ride and we would see them all. We decided to visit Karnac and Luxor first by arriving in Karnac at 6 a.m. before the tourists got there, so we could have a private experience without a guide and a crowd. Personally, most of the average Egyptian guides bored us, since they believed the earth was created six thousand years ago their explanation of Egyptian history appeared uninformed to us.

Delilah and I experienced the colossal columns and statues with our intuition and imagination as we walked around the temple halls and grounds. I believe we were connecting with an ancient part of ourselves, while there seemed to be a feeling of familiarity as we carefully took in the antiquated hieroglyphs. Around 8 a.m. we began to feel invaded because the regular tourists started to enter the temple, so we chose to move on to downtown Luxor and visit the Luxor Temple for the rest of the morning and afternoon.

When we entered the temple grounds; Delilah marched ahead and walked past a group of schoolchildren who simultaneously turned their heads, staring at Delilah while she hiked past. I was the witness walking slightly behind as Delilah forged ahead, not taking notice of the kids passing and staring. It felt as if they recognized her somehow. Just a few days before in Cairo at the open marketplace strangers called out to us,

"Cleopatra! Neferatiti!"

It appeared that Delilah was Cleopatra and I was Neferatiti to the anonymous observers.

Delilah has beautiful, striking facial features that resemble more Mediterranean heritage than her Norwegian ancestral family lineage. Her recognition as a world-famous belly dancer with a Norwegian legacy stumps her students and fans.

We explored the Luxor Temple and managed to venture off away from the tourist hordes and Delilah knew of a small Sekhmet (the lion-headed female goddess) temple off the beaten path. This was quite a treat since the tour guides do not show this temple to people and it has the only known intact Sekhmet statue in Egypt. There are a tremendous amount of artifacts still buried, much more than have been excavated, so who knows, there may be several intact Sekhmets hidden all over Egypt.

We came upon a small stone building with two long blue caftan-wearing guards sitting outside on a semicircle stone bench. They were happy to see us since they don't receive normal tourist traffic and were very eager to show us the temple. We were escorted inside a large dark room with a thin beam of sunlight peeping through a small square opening in the wall. Sekhmet stood tall in her majesty with her sun-disk halo and long sacred sceptre, patiently waiting in the back of the room for her reverent admirers. Delilah and I stood in awe and prayer and felt her power, unpacked our wine, and began anointing the Lion Goddess' chakras and feet. Delilah christened her with wine while I took my essential oils of frankincense, sandalwood, and myrrh and anointed her, following the same path as the wine. I believe Sekhmet followed me home and reinforced her relationship with me after that.

The ancient Egyptian description of Sekhmet was represented by the searing heat of the midday sun (in this aspect she was sometimes called *Nesert*, the flame) and was a terrifying goddess. However, for her friends she could avert plague and cure disease. She was the patron of physicians and healers, and her priests became known as skilled doctors. As a result, the fearsome deity sometimes called the *lady of terror* was also known as the *lady of life*. Sekhmet was mentioned a number of times in the spells of *The Book of the Dead* as both a creative and destructive force, but above all, she is the protector of Máat (balance or justice) named *The One Who Loves Máat and Who Detests Evil*.

Feeling quite satisfied with another mystical, spontaneous, adventurous day we headed back to the Luxor Hilton to nap and decorate ourselves for dinner. The dinner show consisted of belly dancing and cobra snake taming. The belly dancer invited guests to join her and Delilah and I took her up on the invitation. She was surprised when we could match her movements and we added a few of our own. She was unaware of the entertainment the night before when Delilah had stolen the show. She seemed to appreciate our talented company on her stage and was inspired to dance with more enthusiasm than her normal touristy routine.

Then out came the snake tamer with his Egyptian woven baskets, hypnotic flute, and scary-looking, defanged cobras. Of course Delilah volunteered to be draped with cobras while dancing to a mesmerizing flute. I am reminded of the time Delilah owned a pet boa constrictor named Cecelia that she often used in her dance performances. On one occasion among many, Delilah and I had been parade participants with Delilah's Visionary Dancers in the Fremont Pagan Summer Solstice Parade using Cecelia as the most attention-getting prop. At the end of the parade there was a huge festival to explore, and drinking establishments to frequent. We had Cecelia with us and attempted to enter a local brewery and were promptly turned away as no pets were allowed. Delilah pulled out her trusty snake pillowcase and placed Cecelia safely inside as we re-entered the brewery with a concealed snake and proceeded to innocently order beers unnoticed.

The next morning back in Egypt we made arrangements to visit Dendera early in the morning before the tourists arrived. It was about an hour and a half cab ride so we met our new amused Coptic Christian guide at 5 a.m. sharp in the Hilton lobby. I wish I could remember his name because he was so excitedly challenged and honored by our special request. At one point the cabdriver indicated he was taking a left toward the temple of Dendera and a bus load of tourists appeared to be moving in the same direction and all of a sudden the bus made a U-turn and went the opposite route. Delilah and I were very happy to see that and soon we arrived at the temple with no one else in sight. Delilah brought her Hathor costume and video camera and planned to dance while I filmed her. We brought baksheesh to pay extra for taking video equipment into the temple, as this is the normal procedure. The guards waved us on and said it was free today.

Our guide gave us a private tour with his understanding of Egyptology while I videotaped. Dendera is known as a temple to the Goddess Hathor. While our guide imparted his interpretation of the hieroglyphs, Delilah and I imagined what the temple was like in the ancient days by closing our eyes and being silent.

After some time we were led down a narrow passageway to see an interesting glyph that may have shown a sign of Egyptian electricity. It was a lotus flower with a long tube shooting out from the center of the flower with an undulating snake inside the length of the tube, like a florescent bulb. The lotus stem looked like a long electrical cord with a plug at the end. The instant we looked at this symbol the electricity cut off and we were in complete darkness. How symbolic is that? Our guide managed to scrounge up a flashlight and get us out of there.

We found a room that we thought might be a birthing chamber according to our escort. Delilah decided this would be the room to set up the video camera and perform the Hathor dance. She found a discreet place to change into her costume while I set up the camera. Her long white Goddess gown touched the rough dirt floor and looked striking against her skin with her jewelry and jet black Egyptian wig. She entered the birthing room and began the dance at the foot of the stone steps in between two columns. She created this beautiful dance at home in her kitchen and moved as if she were a hieroglyph peeling off a temple wall and coming to life speaking a universal language. Later while watching the film, we noticed the lighting in the room started out in sepia tones; when the dance began the room changed to a blue hue and ended with sepia again. This added a whole other mystical perspective and very curious effect.

The instant Delilah ended her Hathor dance the guards zeroed in on the tripod-held video camera and scolded us for attempting to use it and that it must be taken down immediately. Our Coptic guardian host blocked the guards from coming near Delilah and me, and handed them baksheesh to calm them. Since we had completed what we set out to do, I began dismantling the camera so we appeared to comply with their frantic request.

Delilah remained in costume while we continued our temple tour and still no other tourists to disrupt our private time. Delilah would stand in a corner where she imagined a deity statue might have stood as the sun's rays peered through a small temple window and shone on the imagined deity at the appropriate astrological moment. At one point we climbed to the roof of Hathor's temple and danced to silent music. Soon buses of tourists began to park and we knew it was time for our departure, but not before the new guests were pleasantly surprised to be greeted by a living temple deity as we exited. We got the impression that our guide was as entertained as we were and was honored to have helped in the creation of this day.

Back at the Hilton we took a nap and planned our last day in Luxor across the Nile to the Valley of the Kings and Queens. The next morning we ventured into town and found a little passenger boat for a small price to take us over to the other side. We were told that it would be easy to find a cab once we arrived on shore. After the short boat ride we were greeted by a cabdriver who escorted us to the Valley of the Kings and Queens ticket booth. Delilah went ahead of me and proceeded to have an argument with the man in the ticket cave. She received her ticket and angrily said,

"He wanted me to kiss him before he would give me my tickets."
Needless to say she did not comply.

Okay, it was my turn now. I asked for my ticket, thinking Delilah had established a rule and I would not be treated the same way. The ticketing agents consisted of an old man and a young man. The old man insisted that I kiss the young man before receiving my tickets and I thought, *Okay, on the cheek maybe.* The old man insisted that it be on the lips so I got a little irritated and turned to my cabdriver for protection and said,

"He wants me to kiss him."
The cabdriver looked at me and said somewhat aggressively,

"Kiss him!"
Insinuating it was no big deal, give the guy some pleasure and let's get going. I looked into the young ticketing agent's eyes, refused to kiss him, and demanded my tickets, exactly as Delilah. He reluctantly handed them over and said I was mean.

Our cabdriver gave us a guided tour of the Valley and to our main destination, Queen Hatshepsut's temple. Hatshepsut was born in the 15th century BC, daughter of Tuthmose I and Aahmes, both of royal lineage and the favorite of their three children. When her two brothers died, she was in the unique position to gain the throne upon the death of her father. To have a female pharaoh was unprecedented and probably most definitely unheard of as well. A favorite daughter of a popular pharaoh, and a charismatic and beautiful lady in her own right, she was able to command enough of a following to actually take control as pharaoh. She ruled for

LAURA LEGERE

about 15 years, until her death in 1458 BC, and left behind more monuments and works of art than any Egyptian queen to come.

Hatshepsut created a beautiful, majestic temple placed against an orange rock cliff with large jutting rock formations that Delilah and I imagined may have been humongous chiseled deity statues. The temple itself has the original painted walls still intact to a great degree. The famous Egyptian opera *Aida* has been performed there regularly. On the left side of Hatshepsut's temple is a Hathor temple with a locked gate that leads through an Egyptian tunnel maze. Delilah traveled through that gate and into the tunnel her first visit to Egypt when she was 18 years old. She had a very mysterious experience in there with a silent dark-skinned man in a white loincloth diaper. We were so disappointed that we could not enter after try-ing to bribe the guard, who did not possess a key and there was no way to climb over the gate.

After our long day in the Valley it was time to head back across the river and prepare and pack for our Nile cruise. We said our good-byes to the hotel staff, took a cab to the ship, and unpacked in our new stateroom. Our cruise ship was not sail-ing until nightfall and timed with an evening belly dance show and open dancing. We were happy to be able to undulate again as we danced with the welcoming performing belly dancer and inspired others to move their bodies to the sensual, rhythmic Middle Eastern sounds.

The next day we headed back to the Valley of the Kings and Queens and had another tour of Hatshepsut's temple. It was a new experience being with other tourists and we made some very interesting friends. While cruising down the Nile, we gazed on the shore, looking at fertile farmland, conversing with our fascinating new friends, and I had an eerie feeling that we were traveling inside a protective bubble and were sheltered in spite of our naiveté. This hunch would ring true when Delilah and I returned home from our travels; two weeks later all hell broke loose at Hatshepsut's temple. Fundamentalist extremist Muslims ambushed and massacred the first busloads of tourists in front of the queen's temple. Fifty-eight foreigners, mainly German, Swiss, and Japanese tourists, died that day and not one was an American. I believe the fundamental extremists do not welcome foreign influence. This turned out to be the last gasp in the wave of Islamic militant violence that struck Egypt in the 1990s; thank Goddess.

Back on our lovely Nile cruise we recruited our new friends to participate in Delilah's Hathor dance performance for the evening onboard show. Between the two of us Delilah and I brought enough Egyptian costume paraphernalia to decorate our friends for the piece. Our newfound friends were eager to contribute as well as watch the dance. Delilah donned her most glamorous long white gown, complete with a train and covered in white beads resembling pearls. Not the same white Goddess dress she wore in Dendera, this one was much too delicate and cumbersome to drag around on dirt floors in the temples.

Our four friends consisted of two couples, so we dressed the men up as Egyptian guardian protectors and the women as assistants to Hathor. One of the women did not wish to join us, so I became one of the assistants, removing one of Hathor's hand props when signaled. In one hand she held an *ankh* (the Egyptian symbol of life) and in the other a round brass mirror with a wooden handle and cow bone vertebrae holding the round brass reflector. It was a grand display as our entourage presented Hathor in all her royalty, power, and glory, grabbing the audience's attention to watch Delilah dance to her then husband Steve Flynn's brilliant mystical music.

The rest of our cruise we visited temples along the river accompanied by our new friends and their stimulating conversation. Many times a guide would be included with our temple ticket purchase to explain a boring tale. Delilah and I would wander away from this pest and walk deep inside a temple and make up our own story. Sometimes we were accompanied by one of our friends from the cruise who seemed much more interested in our interpretation. Edfu, Philae, and Aswan were the destinations as we left our reverent footprints in these ancient places. If I remember correctly while in Philae our guide explained his low-frequency interpretation of the hieroglyphs. He claimed that the ancient Egyptians were the originators of female circumcision. Delilah and I were shocked by his comment and began to question him. We asked where he received this information and he said it was shown in the hieroglyphs. We asked him to show us where and he did not come forth. Delilah and I have scanned many temple walls, read several books on Egypt, and have never heard of this before or since. The Arab Egyptians practice female circumcision now and this same guide openly admitted this was done to his daughters. He went on to explain that if women do not have this done their something (mumbling) would happen. Delilah and I got right in his face and asked what would happen? He said something like it would grow out of control. We think he meant the labia or the clitoris would keep growing and stick out too far. I guess I have something to look forward to.

The cruise ended in Aswan, so we bid our farewells to our friends and took a cab to our prepaid hotel to rest. Later that same day we ventured out to the marina below the hotel and met a gentle sailor with an offer to take us sailing. We climbed aboard his sailboat the next morning and sailed off across the big river to investigate more hieroglyphs along the riverbanks. Our captain and his talented rim drum musician companion accompanied us as we joyfully danced to his rhythms under sail.

Upon our return our captain gave us another proposal to sail us to a Nubian village for dinner. He said a group of young backpacking tourists would already be there and two more would not make much of a difference to the cooks. He even mentioned that the dinner would be free to us because it was already paid for. We could not refuse an offer like this, an off-the-beaten-path experience with real Nubians. We went back to our hotel to change clothes and grab a few things we might need. Soon we were back on the sailboat heading to a Nubian village adventure.

It was a beautiful sunset evening sail on the Nile as we made our landing.

Our captain escorted us up a long dirt path to an adobe compound where the spicy aromas of Middle Eastern food wafted through the air. We were introduced to a group of English backpackers waiting for dinner after a long day of hiking. They were in the midst of intimate conversation amongst themselves and appeared not too interested in our interruption. Delilah and I ate quietly close by and were invited to have a henna tattoo for dessert at a reasonable price. We accepted and were quite pleased with our beautiful, distinct flower design hand tattoos.

Our host captain offered another invitation to visit his friends in the compound and play cards. We followed him through a narrow passageway to a residence and received a gracious greeting by two of our captain's friends. The large room looked similar to our male belly dancer's family living room. Adobe walls and furniture with pillows placed around for seating. Our captain did the interpreting between Delilah and me and his friends while we played a card game that ended with slapping the losing person's hand. We listened to Ray Charles as Delilah danced and our hosts seemed to enjoy it. The resident host mentioned that the Koran says,

"No belly dancing."

I asked him if he liked belly dancing and he indicated that he enjoyed it very much. These words spontaneously came flowing out of me to address him.

"When you appreciate art from a place of honor and respect, that is how God speaks to you. He speaks to you through your enjoyment through this dance art form."

The moment I finished these words a gecko (small lizard) made its kissing sound. When I lived in Hawaii with geckos, I was told the sound of a gecko means the truth is being spoken. A moment of silence took over the room in contemplation as I waited for a response. Then they smiled and nodded in agreement with what appeared to be relief. It must be hard and confusing to enjoy something natural that is taught to be sinful, and taboo.

I have not read the Koran, but I do not believe it says no belly dancing. I believe the patriarchal society has misinterpreted, misrepresented, wrote and re-wrote sacred text for their egotistical, political control and this is not exclusive to the Koran.

We lost track of time and enjoyed the rest of our spirited evening visit. Soon it was time for our late night sail across the Nile and for much-needed slumber. Our captain had grown quite attached to us and struggled to say good-bye because he knew we were flying to Abu Simbel the next day and he would never see or hear from us again. Delilah and I noticed something different about our host captain than other Arab men we met and spent time with. He was much less grabby and attached to us bending to his will than most Arab men we encountered. We attributed this to the fact that most Arabs are tremendously pressured by their parents to marry someone they have picked and behave according to their conditioned religious beliefs. Our sailboat captain's parents were both deceased and therefore the traditional parental pressure did not influence him. It was refreshing to be in his presence for such an extended amount of time.

Delilah and I were packed and ready to fly to our next destination, Ramses the Great's Temple at Abu Simbel. When we planned our trip and agreed upon spending the night in Abu Simbel the tour company agent questioned why we wanted to do that. She told us no one spends the night there; the normal procedure is to fly in for a couple of hours and fly out and no one stays overnight. We thought great, just what we want to do, not the regular tourist protocol. We received the same treatment when we arrived at the Queens Tours office and firmly convinced them that we were staying the night. No one would give us a reason why—it just sounded like the routine pattern that they followed and nothing else to it.

We were greeted at the Aswan airport to our surprise by two of our Queens Tours bodyguards. We were not expecting them as they grabbed our luggage and protectively guided us to the ticket booth. We were not accustomed to this kind of treatment and assumed this was a small airport with easy-to-follow guidelines to check our luggage and board the plane; a procedure we were quite familiar with, having done it several times already on this same trip. We believe the travel agency in Cairo was nervous with two women tourists traveling alone and felt very protective of us. Thinking back on it, this was just prior to the tourist massacre in the Valley of the Queens, so they probably did have a genuine concern. In addition we were spending the night in Abu Simbel, the big red flag we were questioned about that no one else traditionally does.

We arrived in Abu Simbel at the small airstrip and took a brief cab ride to the Hathor Hotel that sits overlooking Lake Nasser and a short walk to the temples. When we arrived the last multitude of tourists were leaving to fly back to Aswan with no more to follow. Perfect timing as we entered Ramses' temple and his wife Queen Nefertari's temple next-door in silence and alone. The guards opened the doors and disappeared while we slowly and reverently walked the temple halls on our own.

Ramses was the third Egyptian pharaoh of the nineteenth dynasty. He was often regarded as Egypt's greatest, most celebrated, and most powerful pharaoh. His successors and later Egyptians called him the *Great Ancestor*.

Nefertari was the Great Royal Wife (or principal wife) of Ramses the Great. Her name means *Beautiful Companion*. She is one of the best-known Egyptian queens, next to Cleopatra, Nefertiti, and Hatshepsut. Her lavishly decorated tomb is the largest and most spectacular in the Valley of the Queens. Ramses also constructed a temple for her at Abu Simbel next to his colossal monument.

We wandered around Ramses' temple, breathing it all in, meditating in places, and pouring water as an offering in other spaces. Inspecting the mammoth statues guarding the entrance was incredibly striking. We decided to awaken early and position ourselves at the entrance before dawn, so we could witness the sunrise and its rays lighting up the gargantuan Ramses guardians.

Neferatari's temple was dedicated to Hathor and appeared very different than Ramses' temple. Several different majestic Egyptian Deity sculptures marked the entrance and again Delilah and I were left alone in Neferatari's Hathor temple to take in the ancient meaning and energy in silence. Neferatari's great hall is lined with massive Hathor statues. Delilah wore her white muslin skirt and top that resembled her dervish costume; I photographed her while she spun amongst the enormous Hathors lining the great hall.

After experiencing several hours of being lost in time we headed back to our room to wash up, rest, and dine at the hotel. We took in the ancient view of Lake Nasser from the hotel pool; it was a very mysterious scene across the lake; a sea of desert mounds covered the desolate terrain. Delilah and I easily imagined that the mounds might have been pyramids long ago that now blend in as the natural landscape and are no longer noticed or mentioned.

After our rest we made our way to the dining area and were met with everyone boldly staring at us. We seemed to be the only women in the place and no male escort. We figured they all wondered why we were spending the night and not following the tourist protocol of flying in to visit the temples and flying out a few hours later. Delilah and I were a little edgy, keenly alert, and remained aware of our unfamiliar surroundings being two women alone in an authoritarian masculine culture.

While we waited for dinner a most gentle man approached our table and offered his genuine assistance during our stay. We admiringly fascinated him because we were such an anomaly and he sincerely wanted to know who we were and what we thought. He offered to take us back to the temples this same night. The temple guards were his friends and would allow us to enter after hours and of course we accepted without hesitation and we're honored to be asked. So now we had a male escort.

Our new friend led us along the dimly lit path back to Ramses' temple and asked thought-provoking questions to get to know us. We loved his line of questioning, very intimate and sincere; we felt safe, protected, and uninhibited in his company. He walked us past the temples and straight to the guard's sleeping quarters to a tent nearby. There was no one around to get a key, so we would not have a private night showing as we'd hoped. We opted to climb on top of Ramses' temple and tell stories and dance with our new friend. He was enchanted and enjoyed himself as much if not more than we did.

After a satisfying night of dreaming we awoke before the crack of dawn to watch the sunrise on the gigantic Egyptian Deities guarding the temple entrance. What a sight to behold as the ancient stone sculptures performed their daily ritual with the rising sun as they have for many centuries. Delilah still wore her dervishy white skirt and top as she performed her Hathor hieroglyph dance for the Ramses Deities while I filmed. When she finished we were approached by a French tourist, who praised her dance and asked where Delilah had learned such beautiful movements because it brought her to tears. The tourist said,

"It must be taught and shared."
Delilah let her know that she was a belly dance teacher and would definitely be

sharing the dance. Through her tears the woman acknowledged how special it was for her to witness Delilah's stirring private ritual dance at sunrise in an ancient sacred place.

After getting lost in time again, experiencing the early morning sun upon the temples we walked back to our hotel to pack and check out. We were scheduled to fly to Cairo later and spend one more full day in Egypt before our last flight back home. We said good-bye to the Hathor Hotel and were pleased we chose to spend the night in spite of everyone's objection.

Once in Cairo we went back to Giza on our last day to bid farewell to the antiquated artifacts and structures. We went up to the ticket counter and purchased tickets to explore the area in general as a man came from behind and grabbed our tickets at the same time the issuer passed the stubs toward us. He told us he would lead our way, as Delilah angrily protested and I was in shock by his rude behavior. We followed because we happened to be walking that way and tried to ignore him most of the time and by now we were seasoned and on to con-artist conduct. We were also low on baksheesh and not feeling very generous with strange men who attempted to commandeer our otherwise peaceful homage. We visited some tombs and more ancient wall structures and admired the guardian sphinx again. Our uninvited escort was anxious to see us return the next day and showed open disappointment that we were flying back to the United States instead. He was even more disappointed that we did not offer him much of a tip for his intrusive guidance.

On the flight home we wore our metal Egyptian *uraus* (third eye cobra) head-bands and received lots of attention and lively conversation as we had intended. A man sitting next to me asked,

"What did you miss the most about America?"

I paused to think for a moment and came up with an easy answer.

"American men."

Until that moment I had not realized how much I appreciated American men. I felt a sense of relief and thought, *They just leave you alone*. I was reminded that my Americanized Senegalese Muslim Greo Shaman drummer patiently awaited my return. Now that's America!

What an adventure this was! I felt as if I had revisited an ancient life I lived with someone who had lived it with me. I believe it was an experience to help me remember who I really and truly am and to reclaim my empowered essence.

My relationship with Delilah deepened and expanded as I began to work for her and her husband Steve part-time at Visionary Dance Productions. Steve taught me how to use a Mac computer and since he is left-handed I still use a left-hand mouse. I answered belly dance questions over the phone, booked their retreats, classes, and sold, packed, and shipped belly dance DVDs and CDs, belly dance attire and paraphernalia. I worked for VDP two days a week and built my massage practice the rest of the time. The business training I received at VDP helped me immensely with my own business and pushed me past my refusal to use a computer. I give much tribute to Delilah and Steve for their entrepreneurial spirit, education, creativity, love, and friendship.

~ 11 ~

Let's get back to my beginnings with Peter. I hesitated to invite Peter to the Winter Solstice Feast because I was very focused and preoccupied with the performance. Not that I perform very often, mostly through the years with Delilah and her Solstice projects. I did not want to feel torn and distracted on this night. He would be with me shortly and I would be able to focus all of my attention on him then. He planned to arrive Christmas Eve and began his trip from Boise December 23rd the day after the Winter Solstice Feast. The morning of the feast Peter and I were talking excitedly about how soon it was going to be until we finally met. I was going to wait until he arrived so we could confirm the chemistry before I invited him to a New Year's Eve event. I was feeling quite confident in that moment on the phone and I decided to ask him anyway. I asked if he was bringing his passport. He answered that he had it and I said,

"I might as well ask you now. Would you like to go to a Sex, Passion & Enlightenment New Year's Eve party in Vancouver, Canada?"

"Oh my God," he exclaimed in his deep, masculine, sexy southern accent.

I felt a tickling sensation pulse through my body at his words and thought, *He is so worth the risk of making plans before we've met.*

Sex, Passion & Enlightenment is one of many workshops offered by one of David Deida's longtime students, Satyen Raja. Satyen is a wonderful, passionate teacher who has truly mastered the teachings of David Deida and beyond. He and his wife lead by example and have great honor, respect, and passion for each other. They co-teach the Sex, Passion & Enlightenment two-and-a-half-day intensive. The New Year's Eve party is an extension of that work with all the people who have taken the workshop and their friends. The celebration's purpose is to set the intension of Sex, Passion & Enlightenment throughout humanity. What a wonderful way to start the New Year and no, it's not an orgy. The work is more about feeling into someone, connecting through intimate personal conversation while eye gazing without physically touching; the deeper bond that we may be missing in our busy, distracting lives. I was ecstatic that Peter enthusiastically accepted my invitation and would be my date for the event.

This was Peter's last email to me. He was skiing in Jackson Hole the week of the Solstice, drove back to Boise to pack and head to Seattle.

IT'S NOT WEIRD ANYMORE

My most beautiful beloved,

I spent the rest of the trip yesterday being opened by your love seeing it in all its fullness. It is you I have been looking for to share this orgasmic love of cosmic proportion. I kept saying oh my God! As visions of what is coming were revealed to me, I literally could feel orgasmic waves washing over me as I envisioned loving you in every way possible. It started to snow the last 2 hrs of the trip, which is my sign for blessings. Do you realize how blessed we are to make this connection, to have this love that most mortals can't even imagine. There are many angels this day singing and laughing at the joy you and I are about to bestow upon each other and the world! Must pack now there is this goofy girl I'm going to drive toward today on thru the beautiful snow and deliver myself into you with all I am!!!! My love and blessings are eternally yours, Peter

~ 12 ~

I planned to clean house, put the last few decorations up, and recover from the feast while Peter made his way to Seattle. I woke up late and immediately started cleaning and clearing my bedroom to create sacred space. I did my rituals and sprinkled the bed with Holy Water and washed the bedding. As soon as I started this process, Peter called to give me a progress report. I told him what I was doing and he seemed quite comfortable with that, as if he expected it. As the day wore on we kept each other informed of our movements; he was making amazing time driving. By evening he was so close and the weather report was calling for heavy snow on Snoqualmie Pass, so I told him to just get here. He left Boise at 10 a.m. and arrived at my house at 8 p.m. Not bad for traveling 520 miles on secondary highways and mountain passes with rough weather following close behind. I was running my last errand and wasn't at the house when he called to tell me he was in Seattle. I told him I would meet him at the house and was on my way. As I turned onto my street I came upon a moving silver Prius that had Idaho plates and I knew who it was. I flashed my lights and he let me get ahead so I could lead him to the right house. We parked and greeted each other quietly while I helped him bring his things in. I remained calm since I had rubbed the essential oil blend of *Peace and Calming* around my neck and over my heart.

I made him some tea and something to eat and we began to connect face to face. The chemistry and attraction were definitely there. At one point we looked at each other and felt the same thing. I said,

"It's about time you got here."

Meaning, I have been waiting for you for years. He agreed and we became silent and basked in each other's energy, gazing into each other's eyes. I felt that tingly warmth move through my body again, it was so comfortable; it was like being at home with a long-lost friend. After we talked for a couple of hours I asked him if

he would like to get more comfortable. He hummed,
"Uh huh."
As we got into bed he looked at me and said,
"I'm going to wake up with you every morning for the rest of my life."
I felt my eyes bug out of my head and was speechless. I didn't know about that for myself, but I loved hearing him say it. It was exciting to slowly explore our bodies for the first time, making love and falling fast asleep in each other's arms. My Christmas present had arrived!

Christmas Eve we were invited to my friend Karen's house for dinner. I was glad to have another friend's approval of Peter and have him feel comfortable in his new surroundings. Karen seemed very relaxed to express herself with him. We ate the best turkey ever, decorated her tree, and looked forward to the prospect of waking up with each other Christmas morning.

As we awoke we began to gather the other gifts we had retrieved for this occasion. Peter went first and presented me with this beautiful, small ivory and marble box with mother-of-pearl inlay from the Taj Mahal. He nudged me to open it, and as I did he reached in and placed a wondrous gold ring with an etching of Isis on my finger. He told me he had purchased the ring in Egypt at the pyramids. The woman he was in a relationship with at the time wanted him to give it to her and he refused because he thought he had bought it for himself. He said it wasn't until he connected with me that he knew who the ring was for. Then he pulled out two stunning blue topaz earrings and said he was guided to buy these, back in September, and had no idea who they were for. I was in heaven; this was like a fairy tale. I think I pinched myself to make sure this was a waking dream.

One of Peter's wonderful gifts that he gave me every day was waking me up with a beautiful prayer while holding me tight and whispering it in my ear. Sometimes he said a prayer in the middle of making love. My left-brain was so far gone when we made love that I was pretty speechless and could only moan amen.

Here are two of his love poems:

I Am Me

I see me in a patch of blue in the sky surrounded by gray

I hear me in the chatter and the song of the birds

I feel me in the caress of the wind and breeze

I taste me in the love nectar that flows from my beloved

I smell me in the flower of a woman as it displays its excitement

All these experiences created in eternity

IT'S NOT WEIRD ANYMORE

Always will each moment have its place, freely created, freely chosen

I freely choose now to experience myself in abundance of all things of light and love

To open myself in all forms to experience nurturing one to another

Relishing this richness of all the senses entwined with and being that which is

No part of this self can hide from the other because there is no other only one

Evermore conscious, divining more ways in which to love itself, know itself in a play of total freedom.

The Divine In Me

Imagine with me if you will, a love that brings an interstellar thrill

That you finally found that which is love in the form of a girl

You know you've walked eons to be here now in this place of time

To be with this one special one who is the pure gift of the feminine divine

And oh, to dance in this sensual place goes beyond anything ever called bliss

To look into each other's eyes as you share in the eternal kiss

Come all and be this sacred conduit of love with us

The divine in the feminine, opening eternally to the masculine focus

Now in the now I in the I, beauty, goodness and truth, this is how I see you

That which is unseen dissolving into the seen to be that which is fair and true

So I fall into you now to fulfill our creation of perfection

Oh love look at us now being all things of loving nature, come into manifestation

By Peter Walker

LAURA LEGERE

I proceeded to hand him my gifts, which were mostly made up of the spiritual healing sessions I administer in my private practice. I remember him calling me after reading my website and said he wanted all of the different healing modalities I offer: Raindrop Aromatherapy Massage, 22-Strand DNA Activation, Unified Chakra Awakening, Sixteen Petal Lotus Opening, and Emotional Cord Cutting. He wanted them all. I gave him Christmas Rumi cards with gift certificates for the sessions inside. One of the issues I worked with him on was getting rid of his petrochemical personal care products. I looked through his stuff and replaced them with organic food-based products and wrapped them up as Christmas gifts. The reason I am so adamant about this is I teach people how to read ingredient labels in my aromatherapy workshops. An important thing to remember about using the synthetic chemical products is they build up over time in your body. They put a toxic gunkie film over your receptor sites at your nerve endings that prevent proper hormone and cell function as well as mimic hormones. Essential oils are known to digest the petrochemicals in your body and in the atmosphere. That is one of the reasons they worked so well in the hospital because they digested the chemicals in the cleaning products the staff used to sanitize the rooms.

One of Peter's major health issues was dealing with Hepatitis C, which he contracted in the hospital during a blood transfusion for a back operation in 1986, six years before the medical profession knew how to test for it in the blood. There are four million known cases of Hep C in the USA and who knows how many unknown cases. Peter did not know he had Hep C until 2003. He only knew he did not have his usual energy level after his back operation and it never returned. The doctor he was seeing in Florida put him on Interferon and Ribavirin to lower the viral count. He had been taking these about six months and made a decision to stop using them just before he arrived at my house. His inner guidance (spirit guides) suggested he get off of Interferon and Ribavirin because they said I would propose he stop taking them anyway and help him with natural remedies. The viral count may have gone down with these pharmaceuticals, but it put the rest of his body in jeopardy. His poor liver had just about had it. The drugs had taken their toll and out of the four stages the liver is gauged by, the higher the number the more compromised it is; Peter's was stage three from the virus and the drugs. Peter described going through the dark night of his soul a few months back, where he was feeling suicidal. These drugs are known for that and people have committed suicide while taking them. Taking himself off the Interferon and Ribavirin and removing his poison personal care products was just the beginning. Needless to say Peter was about to take on uncharted territory and not an easy path in his health recovery. It was a good thing we did not know his health journey ahead.

IT'S NOT WEIRD ANYMORE

~ 13 ~

Okay, back to Christmas day of 2006. My sister Ruth lives about 20 blocks direct-ly north of me with her husband, Mike, and two kids, Robin 16 and Jason 14. She invited us over later in the day. Ruth prepared a meal and I brought my famous pesto spaghetti squash dish. Peter seemed to fit right in and Ruth later mentioned how he felt so familiar and comfortable to her. That could be because we grew up in the same place and are culturally familiar. I must admit there is something sig-nificant about having similar roots. I believe there is an understanding that needs no explanation when you have grown up in the same location. The more friends I introduced Peter to, the more they all seemed to know him. The feeling was, *Oh yeah, him.* I believe this to be what some call your soul family. Peter said he had never felt more at home than anywhere else he had traveled or lived. He'd had an astrocatography reading a few years ago. Astrocatography is using astrology to map out the best place on the planet for you to thrive, and his astrocatography said that Seattle was his town. At the time of the reading he was in Virginia and Seattle seemed so far off, he could not foresee moving there. Peter had been to every state accept South Dakota, Washington, and Alaska. He is a Scorpio and Washington is a Scorpio state and Seattle is a Scorpio city. His moon is in Scorpio also and his rising sign is Pisces. Peter is all water and I am mostly fire with sun in Sagittarius, an Aries moon, and Pisces rising as well. Peter is definitely intense as I can be too and thank God for my lighter side being an easy diffuser for his Scorpio moods.

Ruth and Mike asked Peter how long he was visiting. Peter and I looked at each other and shrugged our shoulders. It seemed too early to say anything since we just met, and then there's the feeling that he's here and that's it. As the week wore on we began to discuss what this was feeling like and what plans were necessary. He was going to move in while I went on my cruise with Wifey. Peter called his friend Jeff and his brother Michael and told them about our near future wedding. He did not ask me to marry him directly, I was only informed about this by the phone conversation with his friend and brother; he was confident we had arrived at that and I agreed later we had. We decided our wedding would take place in Damanhur.

We made love constantly until I left for the cruise. We both agreed that we had more sex with each other than the sex we had when we were in our twenties. I was so spacey from all the lovemaking I could barely function on a practical level. It was a good thing that I had plenty of time over the holidays to be that unground-ed. It was fun to be that juiced up over a new relationship. When you're over 50 you wonder if you could ever feel that way again. David Deida and Satyan's work teaches you how to keep that juice going for the rest of your relationship. This was going to be a great adventure, as relationships are the hardest personal growth workshop there is.

New Year's Eve we drove up to White Rock, Canada, just over the border. We checked in at the pink Pacific Palace Hotel, where the Sex, Passion &

Enlightenment party was to be. We swam in the heated pool and sat in the hot tub while I greeted fellow students of Satyan's workshops and introduced them to Peter. My friend Karen, who had us over for dinner Christmas Eve dinner, was there because she had benefited from Satyan's work as well. Peter and I went back up to the room to get dressed for the evening. He looks good in a suit and tie and so handsome. My thoughts were, *Finally after doing this work I can experience and practice it for real.* After the feast was over we paired with strangers to begin intimate dialogue and continuous eye gazing led by Satyan. We would switch to another stranger and another, until we all felt quite comfortable, free, and liberated with one another. Peter even ran into someone he knew from an Enlightenment Intensive he attended in Oregon. Then the dance music came on and we danced wildly with a purposeful focus. Satyan played specific lyrics for us to move to as we sent our focused, loving, healing energy intention for the planet and out into the cosmos. This went on for a couple of hours and after the dancing, there were performance skits that went into the early morning hours. Peter and I stayed up as late as we could, about 2 a.m. We heard the skits went until 4 a.m. What a wonderful way to start the year, putting forth such positive intent with like-minded people.

We came home New Year's Day and I began seeing my massage clients the next. Whenever I was between clients we made more love.

We both wanted to make an offering to give thanks for our union, so we picked a personal trinket symbol to sacrifice. Peter chose to sacrifice his silver Egyptian ankh he wore around his neck and I chose the Shiva lingam with rice, mala beads, and ruby from my altar. He had a ritual prayer in mind from a book he kept close by. We went to Silshol Park that has a beautiful northwest beach to perform the ritual to seal our relationship. We settled on a spot close to the railroad tracks near a clump of trees that meet the sea. Peter led the prayer and gave me the words to recite as well as instructions of when to drink the water and when to toss the objects to be offered into the sea. It was wonderful to experience a partner who could participate and even lead a meaningful ritual with me. Our twofold intention with this ritual was for others to meet and come together in divine union as well as give thanks for ours.

We then tossed our sacred objects into the sea and blessed these offerings for others to find their divine matches for partnership.

Time passed by quickly and soon it was time for me to meet Wifey in Houston, Texas for the Young Living Cruise, January 12th 2007. Peter took me to the airport on his way back to Boise to collect the rest of his things and move to Seattle. Thank God his things only consisted of books and CDs. He told me later that he did not have a good feeling about me leaving on the trip. We had only physically been together for three weeks and did not expect our relationship to be tested so hard so soon.

IT'S NOT WEIRD ANYMORE

~ 14 ~

Okay, back in the Cozumel hospital with Wifey.

The day after my nose surgery my family worked with Julie to figure out how to fly me to the states. They were worried about me having this kind of serious medical attention in a foreign land and they did not want me to make any decisions. In the meantime the word spread fast about my situation and many came to my aid with their prayers. Julie's whole Ashram chanted and prayed for me as well as my huge network of friends and family and their friends and family. The Rocky Mountain Mystery School I attended sent powerful prayers. My mom said the Unitarians, the Baptists, and the Catholics were sending prayers my way. My PGP friends and associates were sending their healing energy as well. It was amazing because I could feel the energy being directed at me and I strongly felt my spirit guides and many invisible helpers surround me. I was definitely well cared for and felt that the doctor's hands were divinely guided as far as I was concerned.

After my family spent the day calling all the air-ambulances and finding out their prices, my sister called and gave me the different scenarios, of which none sounded promising. This kind of transportation is very expensive and we needed to pay for the hospital stay and the surgery before I checked out. The cost of my hospital stay and surgeries in Cozumel were cheaper than an air-ambulance flight to the states. Ruth did not want me to make the decision, but I said,

"I am making the decision right now and I am staying here, to have the surgery."

I think everyone was relieved that now we knew where, when, and no money out for the transportation. Ruth was instrumental in coordinating things at home, fielding all the phone calls from friends and family and keeping them updated on my progress. My sister Ruth is a very close friend and this situation really drove the point home. Wifey called the doctors into the room so we could tell them our decision to stay and they could notify the plastic surgeon in Mexico City.

The accident happened on a Thursday afternoon; my nose was rebuilt that same night. Friday was spent with my family calling air-ambulances to see about getting me into the states to have the major surgery. Rebuilding the rest of my face was scheduled for Saturday night since I was staying in Cozumel. Wifey stayed by my side and kept applying the oils continuously. She was scheduled to fly out Sunday morning and Peter would be arriving then. The nurses, the staff, and the doctors were so attentive to me. I was truly blessed with all the help I could possibly imagine and then some. Wifey made friends with the hospital staff as she spoke a little Spanish and her sense of humor stayed intact. Many of the hospital employees, including the doctors, would come to our room and ask us about the oils as we anointed them. I think we created a peaceful atmosphere in our section of the hospital because the aroma of the oils floated out of our room and into the hallway possibly calming the emergency room. The oils penetrate the limbic brain system through the olfactory bulb and can have a very soothing effect on people.

Many of the staff came to socialize with us and told us about a hurricane they had the year before. It blew 150 miles per hour for four days straight. There was not one leaf left on the island, they had no food or electricity, and many islanders left for good. This devastated the island, so when we arrived they were rebuilding everything. I could not imagine what it was like for the hospital and little did I know at the time that my accident had a higher purpose that was related to this and relayed by my spirit guides. I explain more about this later on.

The plastic surgeon arrived with his equipment and his gorgeous Goddess wife as the anesthesiologist. The room lit up as she entered. She walked over to me, looked into my one open eye, and said,

"Don't worry, my husband will make you look like a movie star."
She was so cute and I loved her bedside manner.

Wifey began to get familiar with the surgeon and his wife so she could check them out. She usually does this by teasing and joking and then everyone relaxes. The plastic surgeon, Dr. Mario Mendozam, did not speak English; so he let his wife, Sandra, interpret for us. He showed us the steel plates he was using to patch my face back together and let Wifey bless them while he showed us their flexibility. Wifey explained to me later that she asked him questions outside of our room so I wouldn't freak out. She asked him how he would actually do the procedure. He said he would have to cut into my skullcap and pull my face skin down to my mouth in order to put the plates and screws in place. Wifey freaked out and told him he could not do that to me. He laughed since this is normal procedure and he does this all the time on people who don't even like their face and voluntarily have it done.

Wifey came back into our room and began to focus and chant that he did not have to cut into my skullcap and pull my face skin down in order to perform the procedure. I waited patiently for a few hours while the surgeon and his wife prepared everything. As I rested I chanted silently to stay clear and positive. I thought about the movie *The Secret* where a guy crashed his airplane and was completely paralyzed and all he could do was blink his eyes. He focused his mind to repair his body so he could walk out of the hospital by Christmas and he did. Thinking of him helped me believe my situation was a piece of cake. Soon enough the hospital staff came to wheel me out of the room down the hall to the surgery room. As I breathed in the anesthesia I kept chanting, *Om Mani Padme Hum* (aum, to the Jewel in the Lotus, hum) until I became unconscious. This only took about ten breaths. The next thing I felt and heard was Sandra tapping my arm as I was being wheeled out of the surgery room. She said,

"Okay, Laura, wake- up."

I woke up to a vision of myself being wheeled out on the gurney in a beautiful flowered dress; my face was completely healed and I felt myself take a full breath from my nose, while in reality my nose was completely packed. The vision was another comforting gift among many.

IT'S NOT WEIRD ANYMORE

Wifey was patiently waiting for me to come out of surgery so she could call my family and give them a progress report. She expected me to be shaved bald on the top because of the skullcap cut. Dr. Mendozam told Wifey that he did not have to remove my skullcap. He inserted everything from under my upper lip, below my eyeballs, and from each side of my cheekbones. Wifey said I looked more normal than she had seen me since the crash. The doctor told her my face would swell up three times the size, so be prepared. Wifey knew she could prevent much of the swelling with the oils and she did just that because I did not swell up any more than I already had.

I had never experienced coming off of anesthesia before and it was the most discomfort I felt during the whole ordeal to this day. My body got cold and had the shakes while my teeth chattered, my throat was sore from the breathing tube during surgery, and I kept spitting up blood and mucus continuously. As I lay in the hallway with a nurse monitoring me, I became quiet and still for a while. I could feel invisible hands adjusting my jaw and working on my face in places. I distinctly heard my spirit guides begin to communicate with me. They said,

"Don't worry; this is going to be paid for financially. You will have a miraculous recovery. This happened because you need to stay here and finish the spiritual work you were doing at the Mayan ruins."

My memory went back to a psychic reading I had three years earlier that I had no idea what to do with. I kept it in the back of my mind and now the reading finally made sense. I studied at a Mystery School beginning in 2000 and was handed down many spiritual healing tools as an Adept Initiate. The Rocky Mountain Mystery School is larger in Japan than the USA. A high Japanese Initiate from the school came to the states and stayed at my house while she taught classes, gave private sessions, and channeled the Crystal Dragon from Atlantis. The dragon told us who we were and what we did in Atlantis and what we were here to do now in this time. The dragon told me that I used to make the alchemical crystal jewelry for the high priests, high priestesses, and the politicians. When Atlantis sunk they all drowned with my jewelry on. The dragon said I was to make a crystal necklace that encircled the whole planet. When this was told to me, I was at a loss for how I would even begin to do this. I just kept it aside until this day when it finally made sense. Now let me attempt to have it make sense to you. I believe the spiritual work Wifey and I performed just before the crash was about an etheric, energetic crystal necklace that would connect with other sacred ancient places on the planet forming a protective grid system. The Mayan ruins are a puzzle piece or necklace piece from where I see things and I am one of many grid keepers and in my case an etheric energetic crystal grid keeper. Further explanation is given in the next chapter.

~ 15~

Let's go back to the cruise ship with the Young Living Essential Oilers. There are many powerful healers, movers, and shakers that make up Young Living. One of them is a woman named Mary Hardy. She seemed to always be near me at most of the yearly Young Living Conventions among a sea of three to five thousand people. The cruise was a small group of 300 Young Living Oilers and Mary Hardy happened to be two staterooms away from Wifey and me, on a ship that has 2,900 passengers. I was relaxing in our stateroom when Wifey came rushing in all excited about talking to this powerful, intuitive woman down the hall. Wifey told me I had to meet her. When I entered her room I recognized her as someone I talked to at the conventions and was interested in her work. Mary told us about vortexes on the planet, crop circles, and an activation the grid keepers can do called the Holy Grail Vortex Activation; a powerful spiritual ritual performed in places of power, mainly sacred ancient ruins. The details of the ritual activation are described further along in the story. She was fascinating and has written several books, traveled all over the world, and built her son a pyramid in her backyard when he was three. We had a very intriguing, insightful visit with her.

The next morning Wifey and I were eating breakfast when Mary happened to be walking by and joined us. She told us that we had the opportunity to perform the Holy Grail Vortex Activation at the Tulum ruins. Mary explained to us how the shadow government (the global elite behind the scenes attempting to control us) have set up a worldwide antenna system that controls the weather as a weapon and keeps most of humanity asleep and unconscious with mind-numbing electromagnetic frequency waves. According to Mary, the Holy Grail Vortex Activation can neutralize this antenna system and protect the surrounding area from its negative output. My whole body felt like a pincushion, which is usually an indication to me that it would be in my highest and best interest to do it. The pins and needles feeling is how I believe I can physically feel the truth being told. I looked at Wifey and said,

"Let's do it."

Wifey gave me the go-ahead look as we said our parting words to Mary. When Wifey was getting ready to stand up and leave she mentioned to Mary that she was from the planet Meledeck (an asteroid belt between Mars and Jupiter). Wifey and I believe we are both from Meledeck before it was blown up. We had two different readings separately from different psychics and years apart that revealed this to us. Mary mentioned to Wifey that it was very appropriate that she hand this activation to us because she held the codes for that planet long ago and had been tortured to give out the codes so interested parties could blow it up. She said it was her karma to provide the Holy Grail Vortex Activation for this planet to make up for the blowing up of Meledeck. She seemed very happy to have given the activation to us and said she was staying behind on the cruise ship to have a massage and a manicure. We hugged her good-bye and were off for our unexpected adventure.

IT'S NOT WEIRD ANYMORE

Wifey and I went to the first info tour booth we could find and asked about getting to Tulum. The answer we received did not sound promising. Tulum was on the mainland and we were on an island. In order to get to Tulum and back it would be six hours roundtrip and that did not include doing anything else but traveling. We knew if we tried this we would not make it back to the ship on time to depart. Cruise ships do not wait for anything or anyone. I suggested we go to the beach and project ourselves to Tulum and do the activation from the island of Cozumel. Wifey agreed and off we went to rent scooters just like we had planned for days.

Back to lying on the gurney and coming off of the anesthesia. I said to my spirit guides,

"So Mary Hardy gave me my crystal necklace?"

"Yes," they replied.

This was comforting news to me because I was glad to know the higher purpose of my situation. The nurse wheeled me back into my room with Wifey and the surgeon came in to check his work. The other doctors were in the room as well and wanted to check if I could see out of my right eye. I tried to open it, but it was stuck shut, so they used gauze to wipe it with a solution and made it easier for me to open. It came open and I could see and was truly grateful. The surgeon moved his finger back and forth above my eyes as I followed. He said,

"Perfecto mundo," and soon they all went somewhere to sleep I hoped.

I continued to spit up mucus and blood and did not sleep at all during the night. Wifey got up to use the bathroom about three o'clock in the morning and I used the opportunity to tell her what my spirit guides said about the situation. Wifey said it made total sense to her and felt like the truth. She said she had written a spontaneous automatic channeled writing years ago that had to do with what my guides told me and said she would read it to me sometime. I have yet to hear it.

Wifey had another situation brewing of her own. She was a host to a soccer-ball-sized fibroid growing in her uterus and still had an amazingly flat stomach for such a thing. It was important for her to get home and keep her ultrasound appointment. Her doctor was very busy and would be unable to re-schedule her for another month if she tried to change her appointment. Wifey was ready to fly out in the morning and made it to her appointment in the nick of time, thank Goddess. I asked Wifey how she was physically feeling with her fibroid. She said after watching how I handled my predicament, what she was facing would be a piece of cake.

As the sun came up and the light hit the room, I could hear Wifey gathering her things to leave. She wrote an instruction list for Peter with pointers and tips of how to take care of me and what was available in the hospital. She's so industrious; I am eternally grateful she is in my life. Her bags were packed and the hospital staff waited outside the room to say good-bye. In her broken Spanish she said she was very pleased to have met them and thanked them for all their help and attention and she hoped to never see them again. They laughed and hugged her good-bye. Our parting words to each other were,

"Let's do this again and go on another cruise sometime."

~ 16 ~

Wifey figured out that Peter was arriving on the same plane she was departing on. She was anxious to meet him physically because she was feeling quite close to him by now. They met for about three minutes and gave each other a high-five and hugged. Wifey said to Peter,

"You are quite handsome, Laura scored big- time."

Then she gave him the thumbs-up and boarded her plane.

While Peter made his way to the hospital from the airport, I had finally finished my spitting spree and thank God for one less thing to gross him out with. I had not taken a shower or been bathed after surgery yet since I was still resting and recovering. My thoughts were, *I look so awful for him.* I did what I could by plucking stray chin hairs I could feel with my hands. This was a new relationship and you always want to look your best, particularly in the beginning, like a shiny new gift. I did not know what I looked like because I had not looked in the mirror since before the accident. I wanted my focus to be on healing and I quite liked my old face. My intuition had no doubts about Peter loving and helping me through this, so I never spent time worrying about his devotion and commitment.

Peter entered the room, came over to my bedside, and was so happy he was finally with me. He looked at my bloody face and head and checked me out a little. He saw blood in my ear and thought I was bleeding from my ear at first. As it turns out the face bleeds a lot and especially with broken bones, so it was hard for the hospital staff to keep me cleaned up enough. I was also hooked up to a catheter and IVs. He leaned down to hug me and I said,

"I am sorry I look so bad for you."

He looked into my eyes with tears in his and said,

"You are like a diamond to me."

I will never forget his words or the expression on his face. It felt as if he was looking right through me and into the core of my very being. What an entrance!

After the excitement and tension calmed down a bit I began to relay what my guides revealed to me after surgery and what we must do after we got out of the hospital. He said okay, as if he did not want to think about that right now, nor question me in my condition.

Soon the nurse came in to help me bathe. She asked if I could stand up and take a shower, as I had been able to do before the surgery. I attempted to get up, but felt weak and dizzy and said I needed a bath in bed. She and Peter gave me a scrub and washed my hair while Peter nibbled on my toes when the nurse wasn't looking and gave me that mischievous big grin of his. I was in the worst condition I have ever experienced and had been blessed with a beautiful, handsome man to take care of me. This was a very unusual experience as I mentioned earlier; I am unfamiliar with being cared for in this capacity and more accustomed to doing everything for others and myself.

The nurse was about to exit, but not before she took the catheter out, thank Goddess! Now we could have some alone time. Peter began to touch my body and complimented me on how intact the rest of me appeared. I had a few large gashes on my right forearm that seemed to be healing quickly with the essential oil applications of lavender and a blend called purification. I had a few big bruises as well, but that was it. He gently began to arouse me and it reminded us of all the lovemaking we did before I left on this trip. It felt good to feel him so close again. He talked to my mom and let her know that the rest of me worked just fine. She got a kick out of that and was comforted to know that I was very much alive.

Peter asked me how long my healing would take and I told him the ear, nose, and throat doctor who sewed my nose back together said in six months I would be ready for a little more surgery.

"Good, then you will be ready to go to Damanhur this summer."
I liked his forward thinking and felt comfort and support as well as a positive focus for the near future.

At some point one of the nurses brushed my teeth for me. I had not been able to do that and hadn't brushed them since the morning before the accident. I couldn't eat either because my mouth was pretty messed up. My upper palate had been put back together during the reconstructive surgery the night before, and the roof of my mouth could not handle any pressure from chewing anything, plus my bite was misaligned. I didn't seem to be hungry anyway. Finally I put myself in front of the mirror so I could start gently brushing my teeth again. I thought the surgeon was very skilled and I was happy with what I saw, even though I did not look like myself and appeared pretty beat up. Given the circumstances I thought the surgery was very successful. My right nostril was drooping lower than my left since that was the side that was half off and there was a lot of scar tissue weighing it down. My right eye was very red and more swollen than my left eye because of the broken orbital bone. I was still bleeding a little from my nose even though it was packed, and I had a smaller gap between my front teeth. Smaller than when I arrived at the hospital. The nurses kept a gauze pad under my nose to catch the drainage. Other than that I did not have any bandaging and still no pain. Brushing my teeth made me feel like I was progressing and more attractive to Peter and myself. He could not kiss me on the mouth, nor get very close to my face. He would lean down to look me closely in the eyes and I would turn away protecting myself because I could not feel my face. It felt as though he would crash into me. I am sure this was just a reflex from the accident. We talked about it openly so he could understand what it felt like for me.

Peter brought all the stuff Wifey and I requested and more. He brought my liquid health drink mix, so I could get some nutrition back in my system, some other essential oils, especially helichrysum, to heal with, and a portable DVD player. He read Wifey's instruction list she prepared for him and really appreciated it as well as got a good laugh. He was also a skillful healer and applied the oils to my face and body five times a day. He layered lavender, frankincense, and helichrysum on my face and gave me a Raindrop Aromatherapy Vitaflex treatment along the spine points on my feet, a treatment he had just learned before he left Seattle to meet me in Cozumel. The combination of his energetic, healing hands and the oils were wonderful. The oils he used were valor (blend), oregano, thyme, basil, wintergreen, cypress, marjoram, peppermint, aroma seize (blend). I smelled like a pizza. Raindrop Therapy can help stimulate energy impulses into the central nervous system and throughout the whole body. It is known for helping repair bone, nerves, ligaments, and muscle as well as clean receptor sights at nerve endings for proper hormone and cell function. It can help bring the body into balance and re-alignment as well as help reduce spinal inflammation and may draw out viruses that can remain hidden in the spinal column and sacrum. It's great with a full body massage when you have access to the spine as well as the feet. Wifey and I are famous for giving this treatment. I have several clients with degenerative spinal issues and they say the Raindrop treatments have helped straighten their spine and reduce and eliminate pain.

Peter was able to lie down with me in my bed and watch some DVDs. He brought a good documentary on *Crop Circles* and I had purchased one from Mary Hardy that I wanted to watch as well. Both DVDs were incredibly synchronistic. Mary had crop circles in hers along with ancient sacred sites and vortexes around the earth. This helped explain to Peter what our next adventure would be after the hospital stay. Peter began to remember that he had unfinished business in Cozumel. He had been to Cozumel two and a half years earlier with an ex and her parents. The parents kept getting sauced, so Peter ended up babysitting them instead of exploring. He wanted to go to a Mayan fertility temple on the island to make an offering and could not get away to do it. When he mentioned this I knew that he was part of the plan to do the vortex activations with me. The timing was impeccable and very synchronistic, and when you are in this cosmic flow you are in the flow with one event directly related to the next event. At this point I believed we came together to do service work as a team. He also said that when he would look at my pictures on my Match.com profile, he kept hearing his spirit guides say,

"Her nose is going to be different."

At the time he did not understand what that meant because he didn't think I was interested in having voluntary plastic surgery. I kept hearing my guides say,

"He is going to help you."

I thought they meant he was going to help pay living expenses. When he walked into the hospital room and looked at my face, he understood what his guides meant about my nose. I used to have a long Native American nose with a bridge and now I have a shorter Meg Ryan nose or Mexican nose.

IT'S NOT WEIRD ANYMORE

One of the points that Mary Hardy made in her DVD was all the hoopla about Y2K at the millennium. She said that the Great Cheops Pyramid in Giza is a huge antenna and the shadow government tried placing a gold capstone on the top of the great pyramid. This would have shut down man's electrical and electronic grid system around the globe and that was the plan; hence the world computer shut-down scare. The Egyptian government would not allow them to do it, so the antenna system was set up instead. I felt empowered to have the antidote of the vortex activation.

Later in the evening Peter and I locked the door and began to get a little more familiar with each other. We learned new ways of touching and caressing since I could not move around much, so we made love very slowly, gently, and sweetly. I was in heaven.

The next morning Peter took my health drink mix to the cafeteria and made me a delicious drink blend with the local fruit. The staff brought his breakfast to him in our room just like they did for Wifey. Peter could not believe the service at the hospital. When night fell we would get a little cozier with each other and be making love and have to stop because the nurses needed to check on me. By the way the door did not lock as we had thought. One night we were making too much noise and the night nurse attempted to come into the room. We stopped and began to laugh and the nurse knew not to enter. Peter would get up in the morning, go to the cafeteria to make my breakfast drink, and notice the staff grinning at him as if they wanted him to know that we entertained them. Sex is good healing juju and they knew it. We had a very pleasant experience for the rest of our hospital stay.

Peter fielded all the phone calls from friends and family and got integrated into my inner circle quite fast. In what seemed like an instant he was welcomed to be part of my family and friends. His actions showed them what he was made of and they approved wholeheartedly as did I.

Wifey called to check on me and said she had to have a full hysterectomy right away. I made sure she kept me posted about her progress. She laughed at us for making love in the hospital and loved hearing about it. She said,

"Look at you, you're face is all smashed in and you have had more sex than you've had in years."

It was so hard to keep my mouth from smiling and my face from moving with laughter.

Her surgery was scheduled for two and a half hours the next day. When she called back after the surgery, she said the doctor was surprised that she only needed to work on her for one hour. The other one and a half hours were scheduled for dealing with scar tissue because of past surgeries in the same area, but there wasn't any. Wifey attributes this to the enzymes called VitalzymeX she took for three months before the surgery that digest scar tissue. Her doctor agreed to let her use the essential oil protocol for the post surgery pain. It worked like a charm and Wifey did not have to use painkiller drugs to recover. She and I agreed that the beginning of 2007 was so intense for us and we looked forward to what was next because it must be gentler and tamer than this.

Five days had passed since my nose surgery and it was time to take the packing out of my nostrils. I was a bit nervous because I thought I might feel pain and had Peter hold my hand while it was being removed. The doctor slowly pulled the packing material out and to my surprise I didn't feel much of anything at all. I could breathe freely out of my nose again, hallelujah! Two more days passed and I was taken off the IVs and given pills to swallow. I was told I could check out the next day, but could not fly home for another week because the cabin pressure would be too hard on my repairing sinuses. I thought, *This was the opportunity to start the activation work at the ruins.*

Peter changed the airline tickets at no extra charge and found a nice hotel for us to stay. We could not leave the hospital until we paid up since they were quite used to getting ripped off according to the staff. The hospital maxed out my credit card and even went over my limit. My mom was trying to wire her home equity line of credit and could not get it to the hospital before checkout time. Meanwhile the nurse gave me an ample supply of painkillers, antibiotics, digestives, etc. to take with me. I left my passport and driver's license with them as collateral so we could leave and go to our hotel. Mom's money would arrive after the weekend and I could pick up my identification then.

~ 17 ~

The hotel was luxurious, with a king-sized bed and all the amenities. The first thing I did was lay all the pills the hospital gave me on the bed. After looking them over carefully I made the decision not to take them. I had my own medicine, the oils. We stayed in bed and kept up our sexual exercises and ventured out for meals and a little exploration. We even went out the first night to the open town square where there was live salsa music. I could not hold still and had to get up and dance. It was good to wake up my body after lying around for eight days.

We made friends with Francisco, a timeshare promoter at the hotel who set us up with our daily free excursions as long as we listened to the exhausting time-share condo promo. We rented a jeep and drove to the fertility temple, San Gervasio, a sacred Mayan center where Peter felt he had unfinished business. When we drove down the entrance road to the temple. Peter said, "This was not the entrance; I know this wasn't the original entrance."

He was not referring to the two and a half years before with his ex when he did not get near the place. Once we found the tourist entrance we began exploring the grounds and he found the entrance he remembered from the ancient past. The original entrance was on the ocean side and had an archway with an altar to make an offering as you entered.

Peter was having a past life memory of this place and could describe the fertility rights of the young women who lived there and vividly described his past life recall of the fertility rite ritual. The bride-to-be was bathed and layered in specific oils in preparation for the ritual. The women of the village gathered around the new bride to help fertilize her womb. It began with soft drumming and became louder and wilder as the village woman danced around the featured young woman. The young bride was perched on top of a well-oiled phallus fixed to a chair and moved up and down upon it to the beat of the drums. The village women danced wildly and moved in a sexually aroused state as the energy kept building. The orgasmic frenzy came to a head when everyone had a synchronistic, simultaneous orgasm and the drumming stopped.

All right, back to the current time. Peter and I performed the Holy Grail Vortex Activation on the altar in the center of the community building ruins. We observed the energy after each activation; in this place no one was present when we began and by the end of the ritual we were surrounded by tourists. Then we walked around to explore after the activation and people seemed to follow us everywhere on the grounds. A little boy about 12 years of age started talking to us as if we were old friends, and his dialogue and insightfulness were way beyond his years. When I experience encounters like that I think on some level there is a kind of recognition from shared past lives or maybe ancestral spirits are speaking through them as an acknowledgement.

Afterward Peter and I drove around the island and stopped at beaches, tanned, and jumped in the turquoise blue ocean. I wore a big straw hat to keep the sun off my face as directed by my doctors. I wanted to be in the saltwater because I knew it to be healing for the other parts of my body, especially my right forearm gashes. We ran into a woman who was an emergency room nurse in the states. She examined my face and said,

"If it has only been one and a half weeks, you are healing up miraculously and doing amazingly well."

She even appeared a little shocked. This was great news and encouraging to me. Many people would confront me about my face while we ventured out in public since it was obvious I had an accident. I would warn them about riding scooters by saying,

"Please do not get on one."

A group of Mexican men looked at Peter and gestured that he had punched me, and we all laughed. After that I gestured how it really happened by simulating riding a scooter.

I enjoyed being in Mexico with Peter and having a little vacation with him. I was able to find some beautiful silver stud earrings for him that I had been searching for during the cruise. The earrings have an etching of King Pacal's head. Pacal Votan was a cosmic, mathematician, peaceful, humanitarian king who reigned over Palenque, Mexico in the Yucatán for 52 years. He was born in 603 AD and died 683 AD and was known as the magician of time. Pacal Votan's prophecy speaks of the *Closing of this World Age Cycle* on December 21, 2012 AD. As this date approaches, we are collectively in a transition phase of the old world dying and a new world being born. Pacal preserved the Goddess culture the longest and you can feel that energy still in Palenque.

I visited Palenque in 2004 with the Mystery School and we set the energies for divine union, performing ritual and ceremony with 34 initiates at the many sacred Mayan sites. Palenque was our first destination. We, the initiates, arrived in Mexico City and traveled to Mérida to spend one night and began our excursions the next day. When we got up to have breakfast with a huge buffet laid before us, we were greeted by a hummingbird drinking the juice from the honeysuckle-like flower on each individual table. The hummingbird kept moving from table to table drinking the nectar as if to be sure not to exclude one. We all thought it was a beautiful mystical sign for the work that we came there to do.

Okay, back to the current time stream. Peter looked so handsome wearing those earrings with his silver beard, dark eyebrows, and hair. We sat down to have lunch and I looked at him and said,

"We've only known each other for a month and already we have traveled to three countries together."
We sat in silence to take that in and contemplate: America, Canada, and Mexico. It also appeared that we were both in Mexico around the same time the last occasion we visited the country; although we were with different people and circumstances we seem to be strongly linked energetically.

We made travel plans for the Mayan ruins of Tulum on the mainland for the next day. Francisco set us up with another timeshare promo so we could go to Tulum. We took a guided tour through the ruins and broke away to perform the Holy Grail Vortex Activation. We found a spot where our guide had drawn an upright pyramid and an upside-down pyramid connected to form a diamond shape, which is the symbol for the masculine and the feminine. It was placed in front of a keyhole structure that marked the solstices, equinoxes, and eclipses. Peter and I thought this was a great place to perform the activation. We faced each other and called in the Ascended Masters, elementals, dolphins, whales, our spirit guides, guardians, and many others and felt their energy as well as the energy the activation creates.

The Holy Grail Vortex Activation

Please Note: This exercise is most effective beginning with the statement,

"With no harm to anyone."

Bring energy to the Earth in a downward direction:

First create a counter clockwise vortex in the center and visualize the downward energy penetrating the top of the apex of a tiny pyramid in the center and say:

IT'S NOT WEIRD ANYMORE

From the point of light within the Mind of God, let
Light stream forth into the minds of Humans. Let Light escend
on Earth.

Create second counter clockwise vortex three feet out from the first circle and say:

From the point of Love within the Heart of God, let
Love stream forth into the hearts of Humans. May
Christ return to Earth.

While these two vortexes are spinning, visualize the energy coming up in the cup of the Holy Grail.

Now reverse the flow of energy and return it in an upward direction. Spin a clockwise energy field six feet out from the first circle and say:

From the Center where the will of God is known, let
purpose guide the wills of Humans, the purpose which
the Masters know and serve. (Send the energy to the
cities of Light in the fourth Dimension.)

Now spin a clockwise energy field 12 feet out from the first circle and say:

Let the Plan of Love and Light work out, and may it seal the
door where evil dwells. (Send the energy now past the sun to
the Center of the Pleiades, which is the galaxy where Earth
resides.)
Let Light and Love and Power restore the Plan of Earth.

The words are from Alice Bailey, a devoted initiate and metaphysical author.

Please Note: this exercise is best done with three people. Three people create a note of harmony.

My note: I suggest calling in your invisible guides to be the
second and third presence if you are alone or only have two
people. Peter and I have been doing it this way and feel its
powerful effect and intuitively know we have been called to do
this work. We invite others to join us when they are available
and encourage anyone who feels a calling to perform the ritual
where and when they feel to do so.

Our tour guide rushed us out of Tulum to catch the bus and head to the water park. Tours have a strict time schedule and can interrupt your flow at times. When Peter and I entered the water park we were immediately greeted by a pack of dolphins jumping and grinning at us. We felt this was acknowledgement for doing the activation. As synchronicity would have it, Wifey called during the dolphin greeting. Wifey is very connected to dolphins and they seem to appear just for her even on the phone. I was reminded of the day we boarded the cruise ship. While we unpacked our suitcases we looked out our porthole and there was a dolphin swimming right in front of our stateroom and this was in Galveston, Texas in a very busy ship zone. We felt magickally welcomed aboard.

Peter went swimming in the people's designated side of the park, while I tanned below my chin and became bored so I retrieved an inner tube, a life jacket, flippers, and jumped in with my big hat. I paddled around, attempting to get from point A to point B because it felt good to move my body and immerse myself in the healing properties of saltwater.

We felt accomplished after the two activations and could go home satisfied that we answered the call to help protect the area from more disastrous man-made weather wars and mind-numbing electromagnetic frequency waves. We retrieved my passport and driver's license from the hospital and while we were there Dr. Amora (aka Dr. Love) removed my stitches. It felt great to see him again and visit the staff briefly.

Peter and I enjoyed our last couple of days by going on excursions during the day and having a nice dinner. We went to the mainland one more time for Peter to snorkel on a beautiful reef in a real Mexican town called Puerto Morelos. This beautiful quiet place had not been taken over by the timeshare condo assimilation process yet. We found a boat to take us out to the reef. I put on a life jacket, flippers, and my big hat and followed Peter through the reefs on the surface. Some of the reefs were shallow and I did not want to scrape my body on the coral, plus it was pretty rough out. Peter seemed very surprised that I had the strength to swim around in it. He kept a close eye on me just in case. I did not seem to be aware of how rough it was. The other passengers complained that they had a difficult time snorkeling because of the rough seas and wanted their money back. I was oblivious to this and enjoyed feeling my strength beginning to come back.

When Peter and I returned to the hotel we packed our things and prepared to fly back to Seattle the next morning. We went up to the ticket counter to check our bags and the ticketing agent looked at me and remembered Wifey changing her ticket because of the situation. He helped her find a direct flight and did not charge her a thing. I remember her telling me about him. He also helped Peter change our tickets free of charge too, so it was nice to meet the angel at the airport. We thanked him and proceeded to the waiting area to board. I took a couple of pain-killers just in case the cabin pressure was hard on my sinuses for the short flight to Houston, Texas. I did not feel a thing and decided against taking any more painkillers on the connecting flight.

~ 18 ~

It was good to be home and start working again. I could not schedule as many massage clients as I had before I went on the cruise. My regular intense yoga routine was no more. I had to find gentler yoga positions to do and lots of sex became my exercise. I didn't suffer too much. My friends wanted to see me and I had so many messages and emails I could not keep up. I learned to let go and just let it be that way. My friend Faye offered Cranial Sacral therapy, my friend Kitty offered acupuncture, my friend and massage therapist Rochelle offered Lymphatic Drainage and massage. Teresa offered her Quantum Biofeedback Machine (aka *Hal* from the *2001 Space Odyssey*) to check my body stressors and give me my homework to do. Fortunately my friend Gayle insisted on giving me colonics to purge my body of the pharmaceutical drugs and help my system get back on track. Detailed descriptions of each of these methods are in the resource section in the back of the book. I took them all up on their offers because I know how valuable and beneficial they are. My teacher Gudni from the Mystery School set up an event called the Raphael Healing Temple and offered to donate all the money to me. My family collected donations from our family and their friends, and my sister Ruth set up a Benevolent Fund at our credit union. The combination of the two donation drives paid off my credit card within a couple of months. I was so humbled by this experience and it was such a lesson in receiving since I am usually the caretaker.

When I ventured out to shop a little with Peter, we ran into a couple I knew from the Solstice Feast and Delilah's creative projects. They recognized me! They did not approach us at first because they thought I was still in Mexico and that if it were me, I would have a cast on my head. I was happy to be recognized. It was a little strange when I would run into people who knew nothing about the accident and did not recognize me. Some people weren't sure it was me and would question themselves, but when I approached them they knew who it was and felt a sense of relief.

The first official fund-raiser to assist in my recovery was the Raphael Healing Temple, a beautiful event led by the headmaster of the Rocky Mountain Mystery School, Gudni Gudnason, bringing down the celestial Healing Temple of Archangel Raphael (whose name translates as the *Healing of God*). Gudni also added some very powerful healing tones that are only heard in sacred and secret temples. Everyone has the opportunity to request something very personal for his or her self. Over 100 people showed up to this event including many of my friends and acquaintances. I was overwhelmed with tears that so many people knew about my accident and cared that much to come. The main comment was,

"I am so glad you chose to stay here," and, "Thank you for staying."
Meaning thank you for staying alive and remaining on planet earth with us.

The last time I attended the Raphael Healing Temple four years before, I requested my divine mate. It took four years but I believe Peter matches the description of the man I was asking for. You never know how much work is necessary for you to do on yourself before the request is answered.

I have been a student of the Rocky Mountain Mystery School and learned many empowering healing methods. One in particular comes to mind that helped with my accelerated healing. The Adam Kadmon Body Activation I received in 2000, having 24 key strands of DNA activated. According to the teachings most people only have one or two strands activated and this is directly related to only using five to ten percent of our brain capacity. The Adam Kadmon Activation stimulates the dormant strands so you can begin to tap into abilities that you have not had access to. In this case I believe this AK body sped up my healing process. In my experience I believe this activation assists you to move forward faster in your life when you take other personal growth trainings. It is not a cure-all or, as Susan, one of the PGP coaches, would say,

"This is not drive- through enlightenment."

There are more details to the Adam Kadmon body and the Mystery School in the back of this book in the resource section.

I was not the only one needing healing care; it was time for Peter to get started with his own healing and cleansing routine along with mine. Teresa worked with him on the Quantum Biofeedback Machine, or Hal, to find out exactly how much stress his system was in. Teresa found several things—the main one at the time were his mercury fillings. Mercury is a binder and his Hep C virus may have been binding to the mercury. Teresa suggested some natural supplements to take for some of his other stress issues. Peter went to a biological dentist who specialized in mercury filling removal and had about ten fillings removed and replaced. If anyone decides they want to do this, it is imperative that they go to a biological dentist. These dentists know how to protect themselves and patients from swallowing any mercury and breathing the fumes. Peter's dentist had a picture of a 50-year-old extracted mercury-filled tooth that showed the fumes still emitting from the filling. After the fillings are removed it is just as imperative to do a mercury detox protocol for several months, if not a year.

I viewed Peter's regular habits of casually drinking alcohol, daily coffee, cow's milk, and smoking his daily half a pack of cigarettes as major inhibitors to his healing. This was very challenging for me to assist without being too attached and dogmatic. He listened to my reasoning and health facts with some reservation and resistance because he was pretty attached to his ways. The smoking was the biggest issue for me as I stated specifically in my Match.com profile that I was not interested in someone who smoked cigarettes. He had not been smoking for months before we met and was still not smoking after his initial arrival from Boise. It was when my sister called and gave him the news about my Mexican catastrophe that he needed something to calm his nerves. Cigarettes produce serotonin and cause a calming, euphoric effect on the body. He kept the smoking hidden from me for a while until I could tell by how much gum he was chewing. I started keeping a close eye out for more signs. One day we were getting out of the car to visit a friend and he said he needed to stretch his legs a little and disappeared around a building. I peeked around the corner and saw him from the back walking at a fast pace and witnessed puffs of smoke coming from around his head. I thought long and hard about how to approach him because I did not want to appear angry and judgmental. We were lying in bed one night and I asked him how he was doing with his new health routine. He said he was getting used to it, but feeling worn out and I gently chimed in,

"And smoking."

"Yes," he said quietly and explained when he took it up again while I compassionately listened with sincere concern.

I sent him to my Cranial Sacral therapist Faye and I gave him Raindrop Therapy massage sessions to relieve his back pain. The pain originates where he had surgery to the right of his spine between his shoulder blades. He insisted on continuing to apply the oils on my face even though I could clearly do it myself. His healing energy in combination with the oils worked well together and he enjoyed showing his love for me in this way. After a few weeks he was forced to stop applying the oils after his hands began to experience a major detox breakout. They itched so badly and he scratched so hard that he broke his skin in several places.

Wifey introduced us to the enzymes called VitalzymeX that digest scar tissue. The same ones she took before her uterine fibroid surgery that cut one and a half hours off of her two-and-a-half-hour scheduled surgery. The surgeon did not have any scar tissue to work around from Wifey's past surgeries. Wifey suggested VitalzymeX would be great for me and I thought Peter would benefit as well. He took them for about two months and noticed his back pain had disappeared where his old surgery had taken place. He said he had suffered back pain most of his life and for the first time it wasn't there. I believe anyone who has scaring, and who doesn't? Would benefit from taking VitalzymeX. It helped shrink the thick scar on my right nostril along with the oils and acupuncture that caused my nose to be lopsided.

Peter would quit smoking and promise me he was through, but it would creep back in again. He would hide it from me until I would catch him. I got to the point where I did not let on that I knew he started up again so it would be harder for him to smoke. I decided he had enough things he was working on because he had stopped coffee and alcohol mostly. Teresa would make suggestions and give him health tips since it's easier to listen to someone other than the one you're with. His arguments about how coffee, alcohol, and dairy were okay for him because...could not hold up to scientific facts and professional opinion. In my understanding of Peter's liver condition, consuming these things was not allowing his liver to have a break and rebuild. I am not advocating he never consume alcohol, coffee, or dairy ever again, but I think it best not to consume them as a regular diet, liver problems or not. In spite of his understandable resistance he implemented the recommendations. I have been amazed at his persistence in receiving a crash course in health cleansing and tweaking.

~ 19 ~

Peter did not let his weak health slow him down much and called his friends Dan and Rio Watson, who lead retreats to Damanhur, and asked them when their next adventure was. He wanted to take me there and have a Damanhurian wedding. Peter was the first to put down a deposit for the retreat to hold our spot and we would see if we could recruit some more adventurers in the Seattle area. The trip was scheduled for June 20th through June 30th to celebrate the Summer Solstice there. Peter and I added a few extra days to include the Intentional Community conference that ended on July 2nd. We were scheduled to depart July 3rd.

During the first phase of my healing process, I began to experience some kind of vertigo. The bedroom appeared as if it was flipping backward or upside down when I moved my head a certain way. I heard my guides speak to me and say,

"This is your optic nerve repairing."

I observed the quality of each episode and noticed that it did not stay the same. There seemed to be a progression of it changing and lessening. This went on for about six weeks and was part of the healing process. With all of the various healing sessions my friends were giving me, this response was a gift because it showed their efforts working. Kitty's acupuncture has helped reshape my face tremendously as well as strengthen and heal the nerve damage and scarring. Her work makes it so I don't need much more surgery. She is also my yoga instructor and has helped me get back into shape slowly and gently. The cranial sacral work with Faye worked wonders, as the plates in my skull have become more move-able so the fluids can flow freely. Many of my plates are fixed and the cranial work helped move the fluids and lymph drainage with Rochelle helped the swelling subside. Rochelle is also my regular massage therapist and has helped keep my whole body healthy. Teresa's Bio-Feedback Machine, Hal, helped reduce my physical body stressors. Gale's colonics helped rid my body of harmful pharma-ceuticals and who knows what else I may have picked up in my digestive tract from my hospital stay. I am in such good hands with my friends.

The donations for my recovery did not stop with the Raphael Temple and my family. My dear friends Delilah and Cynthia (my feng shui interior designer and teacher) set up a tribute dinner and belly dance show for me as well. I was uncom-fortable with it initially and Peter said,

"Just let your friends love you."

The dinner and show was wonderful with about 20 people who came to eat and enjoy the show. Many people were unable to make it this particular night and mailed in donations anyway. It was held at a Greek restaurant with delicious food and the performers were all highly regarded professional belly dancers. Delilah's daughter Laura Rose, Dahlia Moon, Elisa Gamal, and Delilah radiated the Goddess within as they blessed us with their beautiful, delicious, undulating movements. The money raised at the dinner paid for my orthodontia work since I needed braces to correct my bite and the gap between my front teeth. A tribute to each dancer is in the resource section of this book along with an extraordinary channeled story of the *Origin of the Belly Dance* as the dance of creation and is not to be missed.

~ 20 ~

Peter and I have both been interested in tantra as a life practice and particularly regarding sex. To keep it simple tantra is expanded consciousness using breath, movement, sound and visualization to awaken the kundalini. The kundalini is the spiritual cosmic energy located in the individual, coiled up at the sacrum, and can be felt on a physical level when activated.

I directed him to a teacher I have admired for years. Margot Anand is one of the most prominent high-profile skilled tantra instructors in the world today. He surprised me that same day by saying he had bought reservations for her next workshop, *SkyDancing Tantra Facilitators Training Module 2*. In addition we were scheduled to take *Erotic Tantric Massage: The Art of Infinite Pleasure* at Harbin Hot Springs with Steve and Lokita Carter, a delightfully skilled teaching couple the weekend before the Facilitators Training. I thought, *Oh my God, I truly am with the man I have been asking for*. I longed to explore this with an awakened partner, and one who was leading the way was even more exhilarating.

I asked Peter why he signed us up for Facilitators Training and he said his guides told him,

"If you want to study with Margot you had better do it now, she will not be teaching this very much longer."

I was still having dizzy spells at that point when Peter registered us, but by the time we were ready to go the spells had stopped and have not returned. My face was still swollen, but that did not hinder us from pursuing our interests.

We drove south to northern California bound for a Harbin Hot Springs weekend to take *Erotic Tantric Massage: The Art of Infinite Pleasure* through The Institute for Ecstatic Living founded by Steve and Lokita Carter. Steve and Lokita have dedicated their lives and marriage to ecstatic living and share their understanding and experience of tantra through their workshops. Their exhilarating workshop set the stage for Margot's *SkyDancing Tantra Facilitators Training Module 2* afterward.

Harbin Hot Springs is clothing optional and most people go naked to bathe in the springs. It is so peaceful there that the deer and the wild turkeys graze side by side. We could practically walk up and touch them. The massage workshop was invigorating and insightful. To start, Steve and Lokita gave us exercises to get comfortable and familiar with everyone in the class. We were encouraged to bring sacred objects, special clothes, cloth, and mood-enhancing decor for our room and the class. This was very easy for me as I surround myself with these things regularly. We were instructed to make a circle of couples. Peter and I picked our place in the circle and made our nest, as did everyone else. Saturday's focus was for the men to give to the women and Sunday's focus was the opposite. The designated person would create sacred space without the other being present to invite and honor them as the God/Goddess that they are. Lokita guided the men to give to the women with instructions and music while Peter learned new delicious strokes to tease me with. Steve guided the women to give to the men as I learned new ways to please Peter. What a wonderful lead-in to prepare for the Facilitators Training with Margot.

One of the massage workshop couples knew about Damanhur and said they were thinking about visiting there in the summer. After meeting us they said they would definitely be there to meet us for the three-day Intentional Community conference.

Soon we were off to Saratoga Springs Resort at Lower Lake about one and a half hours away from Harbin to take the weeklong *SkyDancing Tantra Facilitators Training Module 2*. Margot's majestic six-foot, physically fit interior/exterior beauty filled the room with light. In her introduction she said that after the Facilitators Training she was taking a sabbatical from teaching in the USA. She invited the students to continue her work, provided we followed her protocol for certification. Margot has a pretty strict evaluation for teachers before she will certify anyone to teach. This is understandable as the material is very intense and can bring up an enormous amount of emotional pain for people. In a formal ceremony in 2007 she passed the lineage of her work on to Steve and Lokita and empowered them to direct the SkyDancing Tantra Institute and its group of licensed certified teachers, and teachers in training.

Margot Anand's *Facilitators Training and SkyDancing Tantra Teacher Certification Program* is a four-week, yearlong program. Those aspiring to teach SkyDancing Tantra have to complete the entire program, together with teaching assignments, personal evaluation, and homework. In other words, there is a lot of time, dedication, and personal work involved.

Out of all my teachers Margot has to be the most relaxed and get-real free spirit. Maybe it's the subject matter, but she is so real and comfortable with herself and others and does not appear to have an authoritarian bone in her body and yet she is an expert in her field. She draws mostly from her personal experience and has exceptional skills to write and teach. Peter and I felt right at home with her even though we were newbies and did not attend the first module a few months before. We were accepted as participants into this training based on our prior experience with tantra and Steve and Lokita's observations in the *Erotic Tantric Massage* workshop.

Every morning we meditated and danced. I particularly loved this because dance is my highest form of prayer. Then Margot would explain and demonstrate the technique we were to teach in the afternoon. There were 32 students; we worked in groups of four and traded being the student and the teacher. Margot and her assistants would observe our teaching ability and give us pointers while we taught. Then the group would give constructive feedback to the student who taught the particular technique. The techniques were meant to build on each other, so day by day we would loosen up more and more.

During the workshop I remember Peter and I had some of our emotional stuff come up that was uncomfortable, although I cannot remember the specifics. We were still in the beginning of our relationship and learning about each other's way of communicating or not. My intention was to communicate clearly so we can understand the pain from other relationships and what we truly mean when we say and do things. Even though words and actions may remind us of an old hurt or pattern, it does not necessarily mean the same thing as in the past relationship. It takes awhile to get to know someone and stop projecting old stuff onto the new person. It helps to be aware of this pattern and take responsibility for it. My PGP training would convey that the reason for forgetting an issue is because it cleared and no longer has any affect. I love the Rocky Mountain Mystery School's definition of a relationship. "A relationship is designed to hold a safe place for someone to be totally and utterly who they are and what they came here to do." I add one more qualification for myself that states, "Even if you don't know who you are, which most of us don't, the safe place is there for you to explore who you may be."

There are five questions that the Mystery School suggests you ask yourself periodically:

1) Who am I?
2) What am I?
3) Where did I come from?
4) Where am I going?
5) What is my purpose in life?

Some of the answers keep changing and that's the beauty of it. There are no right or wrong answers, just the deepening of your awareness of self.

The crescendo toward the last couple of days of Margot's workshop was she invoked her connection to the masters of light inviting their heavenly energy to participate.

Once we established the connection the room was filled with a high divine presence; perfect for the work we had scheduled this day. We danced and meditated on this divine energy coming through for about an hour; I could have meditated all day with this energy—it was intoxicating. This day was for the *MORE* session, *Multi Orgasmic Response Ecstasy,* and it was Peter's turn to receive from me as I had received from him the day before.

Peter has been practicing tantra on his own for years, whereas I just read about it thinking I was waiting for a partner to practice with. I was single for seven years waiting and what a waste of that time because after watching tantra DVDs with Peter, if I had to do it over again I would have learned to be my own divine, juicy, delicious lover. I did not feel as open and relaxed as Peter since I was not as practiced as he. Peter was so ripe for the *MORE* session.

LAURA LEGERE

I decorated our corner of the room with cloth and sacred objects to honor him. Peter and I were the students and the other couple, Lisa and Frank, were our teachers for the day. Lisa and Frank were there to assist in enhancing the experience by verbally making suggestions and holding the energy for the space. In all of the practices the key elements are deep breathing, sound with your voice, pelvic rocking, undulating movements, and visualizing the sexual energy moving from your genitals up through the central core of your body and out the top of your head, and last but not least, good, honest, gentle communication. This can stimulate a full body orgasm that moves beyond and surpasses the genital orgasm. We were told over and over that it does not matter if the penis is erect.

I had Peter sit facing me on our decorative bedding so we could voice our intentions and look at each other with deep penetrating eye contact. We created a sacred energetic protective bubble around us and shared our desires for this session. We stated what we wanted to bring in and what we wanted to take out and reinforced the energies that were invited by Margot earlier. I instructed Peter to lie back as I gently massaged and teased him, all the while lovingly looking deep into his eyes. I began stroking his penis with some new and old techniques as he became quite aroused, and his breath, voice, and pelvic body movements joined in. He seemed to be having continuous full body orgasms after a short period of time. He was in for a ride as the session lasted one and a half hours. Frank noticed Peter's voice needed to get louder because he and Lisa could see a block around his throat. When Peter began to use his voice more he was in such a joyous state. I would ask him after he seemed to slow down if he wanted more and he would smile at me and say yes. When I looked out over the room I could see that there was so much joy and Peter's experience was influencing that joy. Margot walked around to observe and assist. She came over to Peter and could see he was close to exploding, so she lightly traced her fingers from his chest, trickled them up his chin, third eye, and gently pulled his hair on top the of his head. Peter let loose with a more intense orgasm; it felt like light was pouring out of him and filling up the entire room. I sensed that the others could feel it add to their experience as well. Peter experienced an orgasm for over an hour. Margot, Steve, and Lokita were right; it has nothing to do with the penis being erect. When the session ended Lisa and Frank were crying—they felt so happy and honored to witness and be a part of this joyful, sacred experience. I was deeply moved and amazed that sexual energy could be so powerful. Reading about it and doing it are two very different things. Words barely touch the experience. It's feeling the love, joy, and divine connection with everyone and Peter and I were one of the vehicles. This day brought down divine ecstasy for the planet.

Margot teaches all over the world and in her view much of the culture in the USA is based on what she calls the *Anti-Ecstatic Conspiracy*. I tend to agree; we have damaged sex with our religious dogma and when you suppress natural tendencies it can manifest as perverted. The USA is definitely witnessing the perversion of sex, as are other countries that preach the same attitude, *Sexaphobia*.

IT'S NOT WEIRD ANYMORE

Margot wanted to show us how sexual energy is very creative and requested that we get together in bigger groups and prepare a performance the last night. Our group decided to do a skit with George Bush at the podium preaching Anti-Ecstatic Conspiracy propaganda while reporters with funny names like Peter Walker from the Fox Fear News asked George crazy sexual questions. I played Laura Bush having learned some of Margot's *SkyDancing Tantra* techniques. I started moving George's energy up his spine and out his third eye and all of a sudden he changed his mind and joined the ecstasy movement. All the while a sexy angel danced around the room quoting Margot's wisdom and calming the place. This would have been pretty funny if the guy playing George Bush had stuck to the rehearsed script. Just before we were to perform, the George character whispered to me that he changed his script a little. Well, the first part with the reporters went pretty well and then George went off on some tangent that no one could understand and it was hard for me to perform my part of the script. The skit was lost when he did that.

In another performance a group of women in flowing decorative clothing began to dance around a particular woman as they shed their glittery garments and fell away from the woman of focus as she danced naked. I was totally hypnotized by her beautiful movements while she verbally expressed how it felt to feel free enough to dance this way in front of an audience. Her expression moved me to tears.

The show that astounded me the most was the last. Men dressed in black holding long colorful banners formed an enclosed circle with the banner material. The inside of the circle was hidden from the audience and the women in the audience were invited inside the circle. As I entered the circle I was in awe of what I was about to witness. Hidden behind the circle of banners were naked women lying in a circle. After all the women from the audience were inside the circle the remaining men were the audience and this was for them. As the banners fell away, the audience was face to face with a circle of naked *yonis* (vaginas) facing them. It was a beautiful artistic sight of reverence and honor because it was a large part of the healing we had been doing all week. The men were invited to kneel down in front of the closest yoni, say a prayer, and ask for forgiveness if they felt called to do so. The energy of the men and how they received this sacred experience cleared some old pain I may have been harboring about men and sex. Everyone was quiet, humbled, and reverent. This was a very special experience that will be with me for a long, long time, more like forever.

~ 21 ~

Peter had planned our next trip to Kauai, Hawaii with his timeshare program. He said he had to use them or lose them, and who am I to argue with that? I was amazed at all the trips he planned for us. In the past I was usually the one who planned and paid for my own trips. I felt really feminine that I could relax and allow him to do this.

In the meantime I had one more *Contact Talk Radio* show to do. I had a monthly radio interview with Cameron and Divindia on their *Contact Talk Radio* show 1150 AM all last year 2006 and had one last show to do. My accident had postponed it for a while. Most of the shows were about essential oils and health, but I decided to do the last one on Damanhur to see if Peter and I could recruit any more travelers to Italy with us. We were fortunate to have two ambassadors from Damanhur, Shama (song bird) and Crotalo (rattlesnake), who had scheduled talks and workshops in Seattle a few days after our radio interview. The Damanhurians take animal and plant names once they have established their commitment to the community. Their visit was wonderful timing and we were able to promote their events and the retreat. The interview consisted of Peter, Dan, Rio, and me. Divindia and Cameron were the interviewers and have become veteran hosts to a wonderful thought-provoking program they created. Peter spoke about his experiences in Damanhur, while I promoted Shama and Crotalo's Seattle events and the retreat to Damanhur. Dan and Rio answered most of the questions because they were the experts with years of experience there. Cameron was so fascinated with the discussion that he gave us another hour on the air.

Dan Watson, PhD, psychologist and Rio Watson, a Science of Mind practitioner, are international energy healing workshop instructors and integrative healthcare researchers of energy medicine and spiritual psychology. They are founding members and the co-directors of the LaHo-Chi Institute, an international center for spiritual energy trainings and seminars, providing continuing education units for massage therapists and bodyworkers. Dan and Rio teach throughout the United States and Europe and lead retreats to Damanhur, Italy.

Cameron and Divindia are good friends of mine, as well as my massage clients. They have both been very supportive of my recovery. Cameron was so funny about seeing me after my accident. When he heard that I had seven steel plates and 34 screws holding my face together, he imagined them to be on the outside of my face. I told him I was not the Bride of Frankenstein; he just looked relieved and laughed.

Peter and I attended all of Shama and Crotalo's events with flyers of Dan and Rio's retreat to Damanhur to hand out. We would be given a few minutes to introduce the trip and give out the flyers. Several people said they came to the event because they heard us on the radio or received an email from me and wanted to know more. A few friends said they were very interested in going with us, but no one gave a deposit to confirm their spot.

I felt the most captivating event was the *Lost Ancient Civilization of Atlantis*. Crotalo told us the true story of the founder of Damanhur, Falco's time travel through a portal to Atlantis in the early 1980's. Falco asked a friend who was a brilliant artist with a photographic memory to accompany him because cameras and video equipment would not be practical for time travel. I am not sure how the invitation to Atlantis came about, but Falco and his companion were greeted when they reached their destination. Crotalo told us about their three-day tour while he showed us the artist's paintings of the experience. One painting depicted the different shaped cities, with the capital being circles with motes surrounding each circle. The innermost circle was where a sacred temple resided where everyone in those days were invited to rejuvenate, cleanse themselves, and state their dreams and intentions. The other cities were shaped like a star, a spiral, and a pyramid. Another picture showed the buildings to be humongous and people like us appeared so tiny up against the architectural structures. The architecture seemed to have a Mayan quality to it in places and Egyptian in other areas with lots of gold and copper metal motif. Everything appeared decoratively detailed and elaborate, including the clothes. The most impressive painting to me depicted three gigantic statues. The one in the front was definitely an alien and very old because it was being repaired from age decay. The statue behind the alien looked like a very fit male and the statue behind the male was a beautiful female holding her arms just above her head and holding an airport-landing pad. You could see high-tech ships taking off and landing, no runway needed. Somehow I came to the realization that Damanhur was an Atlantian Mystery School during Crotalo's presentation and had this confirmed by the Damanhurians during my visit there. Interestingly enough the place Shama and Crotalo were invited to give their workshops in Seattle were at the Pacific Northwest Rocky Mountain Mystery School headquarters.

Out of all the info Peter and I put out to recruit a few more people to accompany us on our retreat, one person signed up. Roxanne heard us on the radio and was unable to make it to any of Shama and Crotalo's events, but said she felt catapulted to come on the actual retreat. This would be her first time leaving the country and she thought it was time since she was over 50. Peter and I were glad she could come and share a very new experience together. Roxanne and I have known each other through the healing community, so she was a friendly, familiar colleague and sometimes my massage client.

~ 22 ~

Five weeks after our tantra teacher training, Peter and I landed in Kauai the beginning of May. We brought the vortex activation ritual and made specific plans of where to perform it. My friend Cynthia lived on Kauai and gave us tips and places to visit. She told us about a Hindu temple that houses a 700-pound single-pointed crystal. We knew the vortex ritual belonged there for sure. This trip was the first real vacation I can remember ever taking for myself. I usually travel with groups to do specific spiritual work or take workshop intensives. Come to think of it this trip was not devoid of spiritual work, I seem to take it wherever I go. I cannot remember when I didn't have a strict schedule to stick to when I travel. Peter and

I relaxed, swam, tanned, and made love most of the time. It was extremely hot midday and we would both practically pass out by 2 p.m. We took a nap every day about then since we had no air-conditioning, just ceiling fans.

We drove around the small island looking for the next deserted beach to lie on; they were everywhere. The Hindu temple with the gigantic crystal gave tours once a month on Fridays and we happened to be on the island then. We arrived at the gazebo meeting area in the morning for the first tour and waited for the others to finish gathering. Our guide brought us to the entrance and explained the different Hindu Gods that guided our way along the path. A humongous banyan tree that covered what seemed like a half acre towered over the entryway to the temple. A banyan tree is like a huge octopus and has tendrils and tentacles that keep going and going and going, covering lots of earth. We arrived at the main temple that houses the 700-pound single-pointed crystal, meditated, and paid our respects. Then we were taken to the main industrious project. The San Marga Iraivan Temple is hand-carved and shipped piece by piece from India and assembled by the monks who live in the complex. The project has been going on for almost eight years with another estimated six or seven more to go. You can hear the monks chiseling away all day. This is a form of meditation and energy input for the temple from the monks.

Peter and I were standing in a large circle of people on the tour at the construction site as he leaned over to me and whispered,

"There's my ex standing over there."

It took a minute for me to comprehend what he said. I did not want to stare because I thought she surely saw Peter and may be uncomfortable. This was the same ex he had been with in Cozumel with her parents. She did not seem to acknowledge or recognize him since he looked quite different than when they were together. He was growing his hair long and was clean-shaven. He had short hair and a beard for 25 or more years, so he looked very different. I asked him if he wanted to greet her and he said no since it was a difficult relationship and he felt peaceful in the moment and she appeared at peace as well. We thought how interesting we would see her this far away from our home in Seattle and her home in South Carolina and among all the islands we could have picked. I suppose *it's not weird anymore* applies here too. She and her male companion walked up to a platform with a statue of Lord Shiva overlooking the complex, bowed, and paid their respects. Peter and I waited until they left and we stepped onto the platform and performed the Holy Grail Vortex Activation at Shiva's feet, a definite power spot.

We drove away from the temple grounds and came upon an ancient Hawaiian village. We decided this was another good place to perform the activation. We found the main central altar, completed the ritual there, and a brilliant male peacock walked right up to me dragging his gorgeous half-opened tail behind him. Many times I have witnessed animals acting unusual after carrying out spiritual work. It's always a good sign and a thank you.

We had one more place to visit and that was the breathtaking Waimea

Canyon. Mark Twain called it the Grand Canyon of Hawaii and if you've been there you know what he means. It is as spectacular and majestic as the Grand Canyon in every way. Then we drove to overlook the Napali Coast, the west side of the island, and found a place to do the activation ritual while thick fog rolled in and out. Hollywood filmed *Jurassic Park* there; a great setting with the lush deep green valleys and steep switchback trails. We felt accomplished performing the activations in Kauai to protect the island and hopefully the other islands as well. Many esoteric writers state that Kauai was a major point in Lemuria (the civilization before Atlantis) and there are large crystals deep in the ocean around the island.

Our last day on the island I decided I was healed enough; after all it had been three months, so we rented snorkel gear and headed for the beach in front of our condo. The mask seemed to fit and felt comfortable. I swam out to deeper water and dove down to get a closer look at the coral and tropical multicolored fish. I've experienced much richer and better places to snorkel, but I enjoyed moving my body and having it engulfed by the saltwater. Little did I know then that diving down and putting pressure on my face would cause a problem that showed itself a few days later. That night my collarbone area became very sore on both sides. My first thought was, *Maybe I am sore from swimming*, but it didn't quite feel like that kind of soreness.

~ 23 ~

We were ready to fly home and plan our next trip to Damanhur and get ready for the Summer Solstice Parade in Fremont (the center of the universe), a neighborhood in Seattle. In the meantime Peter and I were finding out about each other's emotional state, moods, triggers, and quirks and thank Goddess for PGP. The skills I have learned through the program have helped our communication immensely. It was so easy for me to admit my part in an argument as well as ask better questions to help understand on a deeper level what we make things mean. Learning to own our projections is a big piece to be conscious of and rare to find someone willing to do it. Peter continues to thank me for aspiring to be self-aware. I am grateful to him for being willing to take the time to understand and contemplate what is really going on in a heated discussion or disagreement. Sometimes we let it go and are finished so fast we can't remember what the argument was. There is definitely plenty of healing taking place for us both. I love being with someone who can truly appreciate communicating like this. I just love him.

I am reminded of a man I dated for a brief moment in time from Match.com before Peter began to connect with me. Communication was very difficult because every time he asked a question and I did not give him the answer he wanted, he would blast me with negative projections. I felt as if I was a disobedient actor who could not telepathically learn my lines in his play or movie he perceived. We all project to different degrees; the trick is to be aware that we do it and sometimes we may catch ourselves.

Peter has had a tendency to be critical of people in general. I have noticed this tendency in many men, especially since working in a blue-collar job. My first husband criticized others as well and after I drew it to his attention for two years he finally stopped. With Peter I would ask him questions like,

"What if people do not think and have the same reflexes as you do?"

"Why spend time and energy complaining and being negative?"

He seemed to have calmed the complaining way down and mentioned that he could hear me in his head telling him to *stop whining*. His other irritating trait was to act like I am in his way in the kitchen instead of verbally negotiating with me or just waiting until I finish. I blew up with him on that one and since then he has shifted that behavior. I irritate him in his perception by asking too many questions even though he respects it in the long run. From my PGP it's all about questions in order to have a clearer understanding, better communication, and a reality check. In my observation people become irritated with questions about their thoughts and actions because there are some things they do not want to admit to themselves. There are times when I get angrily triggered and lose it, but I can always be reasonable after the initial blowup and apologize for my outburst. I also make a point to stick to the issue and subject at hand and not bring the past into it. With my PGP skills I contemplate where the trigger originated and what I made it mean. I am a work in progress, and a relationship is a great way to see your reflection.

I get a kick out of listening to Peter take a shower. He sounds like he is having an orgasm; in fact when he bites into a delicious morsel of food he makes orgasmic sounds and when he appreciates Mother Nature he expresses sounds of pleasure. I love that he feels free to listen to loud music while singing and sometimes dancing to it in our house. I also appreciate that he can make all kinds of birdcalls in our backyard, either teasing birds and confusing them or creating a symphony with them. He is an awesome cook and grills outside almost every night all year long, even in the dead of winter in adverse weather conditions.

We were home from Hawaii just two days when I made a startling discovery. I was massaging my clients and as I hugged one of them good-bye, I felt my right breast was extremely sore. I checked and felt a very large hard sore lump above my right nipple toward my heart. It was the diameter of a tennis ball. My first thought was, *Wow, this is the first time I have ever experienced anything like this, now I know what so many women are talking about.* I immediately started applying frankincense and lavender every three hours and shrunk it to a pea size in a day and a half. My other thought was, *I now know what so many women tend to do when they feel a lump.* I have witnessed women panicking as they hand themselves over to allopathic doctors who cut off their breast, fill them with poison drugs that compromise their immune system, as well as other systems, and radiate and cook their insides. True knowledge is power and I felt empowered by this experience. I kept applying the oils and it disappeared within a week.

IT'S NOT WEIRD ANYMORE

This is my hypothesis of what I think caused the lump. Normally the natural skull plates are moveable so the fluids can flow freely. My skull plates are fixed and are not flowing normally, so my lymph system is compromised. When I plunged underwater, I put a great deal of pressure on my skull plates and began to feel the lymph system blockage in my collarbones since this is a major lymph area. This traveled to my breast area where there is less oxygen to move the congestion along and caused the lump. This experience showed me how an accident can cause many more health problems. I feel I must state this again. I am so grateful for all of the wonderful healers and teachers in my life as they prepared me so well for my recovery.

Here is a tip about breast problems. Studies have shown that the breasts receive the least amount of oxygen in the body because of the fatty tissue. When we apply petrochemical personal care products under our arms, hair, and face everyday on top of a bad diet the congestion builds in the breasts and can cause cysts and tumors. Add a tight or underwire bra to restrict the flow and there you have it. Don't take my word for it though, and please do your own research.

Okay, one more health tip. Regular pop and diet pop are some of the worst offenders for damage to the body. Artificial carbonation hardens the cells from absorbing any nutrients and pulls calcium out of the bones. Diet pop has aspartame in it and is a neurotoxin. One of my massage clients developed Lou Gehrig's disease, where the myelin sheath that covers the nerves starts deteriorating and causes the loss of motor function in the body. He studied everything he could to understand how and why he developed the disease. Out of all the information he gathered, he concluded that he got it from consuming 64 ounces of diet pop a day for 20 years. He was a baseball player and was losing motor function in his hands and arms. Ball games are notorious for promoting the consumption of pop and junk food that can cause all kinds health problems.

Okay, back to my health regimen and continued facial corrections with acupuncture and the oils as well as preparation for orthodontia braces. I was directed to a little room with a chair that was surrounded with a big metal contraption. The woman taking the X-rays had me move my head this way and that way. She asked me small-talk questions that she did not seem to really hear or care about the answer. When she was finished she instructed me to sit in the waiting area while she made sure the pictures met her specifications. A few minutes passed and she came rushing out into the waiting area with one of the doctors. They both were astonished at my x-rays and took me in the back room where my pictures were lit up for me to explain to them what had happened. Oh my God! I could see all of the plates and screws. Kind of eerie looking at them all, explaining it to strangers while I myself had not had this close of a look. I got the impression they had never seen anything this severe before. They were amazed at what I looked like because it had only been six months. I told them about the oils and all the other treatments I received and they both appeared humbled and honored to be in my presence.

~ 24 ~

Delilah was planning and working diligently as always to put together a stellar performance piece for the Summer Solstice Parade. This was her biggest parade project to date and she has many under her belt. She recruited 200 men and women to be ancient Egyptians and build a pyramid in the middle of the main square in Fremont, aka the center of the universe. We dressed as winged Isis', Egyptian Gods and Goddesses, belly dancers, and masons all dancing and parading in a choreographed maze. Peter and I became masons since it was the easiest and most needed position. We came into the project late because we thought we would be in Damanhur by then and celebrate the Solstice there. As it turned out the Fremont Arts Council had the parade five days before the actual Solstice so it would fall on a Saturday. It was scheduled June 16th, four days before we flew to Italy. I was extremely pleased that Peter and I could do this together because I love being involved in Delilah's projects and dressing people up. Peter enjoyed being in costume and playing his part. He's almost like having a girlfriend because he lets me dress him up and add makeup too. This was another milestone in our new relationship for me because I longed for a partner to enjoy this with.

We rehearsed for the parade in an enormous airplane hangar at an old military base on Lake Washington. It was amazing to see everyone together all at one time. I saw so many friends and acquaintances I had no idea were in the event, and it was a miracle if I saw them again through the large maze of parade participants. Delilah had an architect and carpenters build a template for the pyramid and place it on rollers as a parade float. The blocks were made of white cardboard and had Velcro on the back to attach to the template. The masons carried the cardboard blocks in varying synchronistic positions as we marched to a drumbeat. It was archetypal, majestic, mystical, mythical, magickal, and fun. Peter and I wore the assigned mason costume attire; white skirt, bare chest for Peter, black-and gold-striped headdress, jewelry, and Egyptian makeup.

The day of the parade we met up two hours before curtain call. The official procession began at noon, so we arrived at 10 a.m. as recommended by Delilah. Everyone showed up plus a few extras. Getting in line, visiting, and taking pictures was most entertaining because when you are in the parade you don't see the parade. I gave the camera to Peter and he took many pictures of the beautiful women, mostly half naked or all naked, none of whom were in our procession. Some in our group had beautiful detailed Egyptian God and Goddess costumes. Sekhmet, Bastet, Nut, Anubis, and Delilah was Queen Hatshepsut with a beard. The beard signifies that queen Hatshepsut was as powerful as a king. One week later Egyptologist's found Hatshepsut's mummy and claimed it was the biggest find since King Tut. When Delilah creates a performance piece it seems to be connected with actual events in our lives and this appears to be a regular occurrence when working with her. She truly fascinates me and I love playing a part in her creations.

IT'S NOT WEIRD ANYMORE

I feel it's appropriate to insert one of Peter's meaningful poems, which was inspired by a total lunar eclipse with an Egyptian theme.

Oh Silvery Moon

Oh Silvery Moon that rides the night

That is the manifestation of Isis Light

See how you draw in the love of Osiris

The masculine's love for you lights you with kisses

His divine light races its way across space so that it may experience the union

made divine by creation

He only knows his love by this union completed

Even during a total eclipse he lights you in red as by the earth his light slips

We are masculine and feminine, sister loving brother, opening ourselves to this

love is the way

To bring bliss and joy and have it stay

It is so easy, like light flows through space

Love comes like this to bless the human race

So thank you, oh thank you, oh Silvery Moon, for receiving the Sun's love and

showing the tune

To sing a song that has come from eternity

Let us now play and dance in these bodies of beauty

By Peter Walker

Spectators had their pictures taken with us, so who knows how many family albums Peter and I are in. There were somewhere around one hundred thousand parade watchers; the crowd gets larger and the route grows longer every year. The rules are no advertising, no motorized floats, and no animals. There are many, many beautifully painted naked bicyclers as unofficial floats since they cannot register legally, but they are there every year. Years ago the cops used to give chase and tried to arrest or ticket them, but could never catch the rascals. This chasing put the crowd in danger and there were a few accidents, so finally the cops called a truce and allowed the bicyclers to parade around freely. Many of the cyclers are painted so well it's hard to tell they are naked. One year a guy painted his body to look like a police uniform as he ticketed the spectators. Someone made a float that had a naked bicycler and a cop ticketing him with the heads cut out so you could place your head in the cutout and have your picture taken. Artists are so much fun to play with.

At noon the whistle blew and we began our procession. Some people in the crowd recognized me and got my attention as I danced/walked by. Our group was definitely the largest and the most memorable. The crowd kept repeating,

"Build it, build it, build it," and we the masons carried our pyramid blocks to the center in the square to do just that.

Since the route was so long and many parade watchers were not anywhere near the center in the square, sadly they would not see the building of the pyramid. My friend Barbara kept the masons in line with her fetish whip. She would ask the crowd if they thought me or Peter or someone else was doing their job and the crowd would say,

"No!" and she skillfully whipped us into submission.

The parade ended in Gas Works Park, so we rebuilt the pyramid and left it standing there. There was lots of free food, entertainment, and picture taking for the parade performers in the park as a reward. I heard people for days after the event say that our procession had the best performance appeal and the most organization. What a wonderful sendoff to Italy to continue celebrating the Solstice.

~ 25 ~

Peter and I felt the significance of the Solstice Parade and the connection to our trip to Damanhur in a few days. We flew for what seemed like two days and arrived in Italy on June 21st, the actual Summer Solstice date. My lymphatic system was clogged from being seated for that long; I could not see my ankles because they were so swollen. A resident of Damanhur greeted us with a van at the Turino airport, to drive us an hour north into the foothills of the Alps. He told us his animal name in English was Sparrow. As I mentioned before the Damanhurians take animal and plant names when they have belonged to the community for a period of time. They let the names come to them in visions or dreams and present the names to the council for review. The council decides if the names are suited for them or not. I believe most keep the names they have envisioned themselves with.

Damanhur means *City of Light* and was an ancient Egyptian city. It was envisioned and founded by Oberto Airaudi, aka Falco, in 1978. He had his first vision of this happy, prosperous, productive, progressive spiritual community when he was 12. He was a very unusual child to say the least. When he was in his early twenties he and 14 others created the foundation of Damanhur. They began digging out the inside of a mountain at the foothills of the Swiss Alps to build these amazing beautiful temple rooms. This was done in secret for 20 years since there were no laws against it, but had they asked permission the temples would never have been built. Ninety percent of Italy is Catholic and this kind of behavior is not understood. The amateur artisan temple diggers dug one bucket at a time by hand and spread the dirt all over the countryside without showing a questionable pile of dirt. They were bank tellers, gas station attendants, teachers, grocery clerks, etc. by day and moonlighting temple diggers and stained-glass mosaic artists at night.

Peter had someone specific in mind to marry us. He said we would wait and talk to Dan and Rio and find out when the most appropriate time and place to have the ceremony would be.

We met up with the rest of our group of 14 retreaters, including our one and only recruit from Seattle, Roxanne. We then received instructions from our guides, Dan and Rio, about the plans for the next few days. Our group was scheduled to celebrate the weeklong Summer Solstice with the Damanhurians and visitors from other countries in the underground temple. We were to spend the night of the 23rd inside the underground temple room of the Hall of Mirrors and have access to the other rooms during the night. The 22nd we spent preparing and clearing ourselves by walking the labyrinth above the underground temple. After the labyrinth cleansing process we were invited to tour the elaborate underground temple rooms. We admired the artisan's creation of this magnificent feat as it prepared us for our overnight stay.

The Hall of Mirrors is dedicated to the sky, the air, and light. It has the largest Tiffany stained-glass cupola in the world. The cupola represents solar energy, strength, and life. The symbols are expressed in signs of the ideogrammatic language, which recreates the movement of animals. The serpent is considered an ancient symbol of knowledge. Access to the other rooms can be reached by descending several steps. Each of the rooms contains one of the four altars dedicated to the elements, air-ether, earth, fire, and water.

Our sleeping quarters were in the upstairs of the visitor center and we awoke every morning to a full family-style breakfast with fresh cappuccino, organic homegrown chicken eggs, muesli, yogurt, and toast and not the usual Italian continental breakfast fare. Dan and Rio gave us our daily itinerary and any changes that needed to be made during our breakfast morning ritual. I do not usually drink coffee or consume much dairy, but you know how the saying goes, "When in Rome." Damanhur raises all their own animals, grows their own vegetables, and makes their own cheese, yogurt, milk, gelato, and wine and I was game to consume it all. Little did I know at the time that I would learn a big lesson about that kind of diet.

The night of the 23rd our retreat group drove to the temple entrance and were greeted by many people from 15 other countries that we joined on this very special night. A beautiful Italian man named Orangutan, and yes it is the name of the primate, led our evening and all-night ritual in the Hall of Mirrors. We carried our sleeping gear into the underground temple and picked a spot to nest. The sleeping mats were a quarter-inch thick and lay on a cold concrete floor. I knew I would not sleep much this night.

Orangutan led us to stand in a circle and greet one another as we shared where we were from. He instructed us to turn around and look into the mirror and find ourselves. He suggested we dance with ourselves, looking into our own eyes and connecting with the other images of ourselves that reflected in all the mirrors. I found myself in eight different reflections and performed the sacred dance to myself that I was taught the day before in preparation to enter the temple. After a while Orangutan instructed us to turn around and form a circle holding hands and we could see eight different circles in the mirrors—it was magnificent! Strong emotions flowed through me while I connected with the others and myself through the mirrored reflections.

Next we were to lie down and meditate until we received further directions. I stuck to my internal chanting mantra of *Om Mani Padme Hum* to keep my mind busy on something useful and positive as I had done in the Mexican hospital. Soon we were asked to move about the temple and experience the rooms in whatever way was appropriate as long as we were quiet and did not disturb anyone.

I made my way through the narrow passageway to the Blue Temple, where a blue sphere with some kind of alchemical liquid resided. The Blue Temple is a small round room with a beautiful naked Goddess (the tarot card *The Star*, the sign of practical idealism) mosaic on the floor with a secret stairway that unfolds from between her legs and leads to the Hall of Water. I joined others as we sat quietly and meditated on the sphere. I continued the chant in my head so I could remain focused because if I didn't I felt that my mind would be too busy analyzing everything.

The Blue Temple is the oldest hall, and is used for meditation on social matters by the Guides of the Federation of Damanhur, as a place for inspiration and reflection. For inspirational use there is a throne in terra-cotta, placed in an alcove in the wall, from which one can meditate upon the large blue sphere.

I descended down the stairway to the Hall of Water to have a look and feel. This hall is dedicated to water and the feminine principle, and is in the shape of a chalice, symbol of receptivity, offering, and a capacity to welcome. Blue is the dominant color, and the neon lights hidden behind the cupola diffuse and soften the light creating a marine atmosphere. The chalice is represented by the shape of the wall and the portal, which is in front of the present entrance to the hall: seven steps lead to a window dedicated to the moon (a typically feminine element) fashioned in Tiffany and cold-painted glass; characteristic of Damanhurian glass windows. There is an indigo blue sphere on a pedestal. On the walls selfic schemes are painted (selfica is the study of the interaction between metals, spirals, and energetic fields that encircle the Earth). The hall is a genuine, authentic library, containing written texts in 12 extremely ancient alphabets. Serpent-dragons executed in gold leaf indicate the flow of the synchronic lines in the hall. Synchronic lines are energy-rivers that surround the Earth and link it to the universe. These energy flows are able to catalyze the great forces present in the cosmos and can modify events, carry ideas, thoughts, and moods, thereby influencing all living creatures. There are more synchronic lines that intersect in Damanhur in these temple halls than any other place on the planet, except somewhere in Tibet that the Red Chinese occupy and is not accessible. Falco searched all over the world for the highest concentration of these intersecting lines and found that he was born within 20 miles of them. He knew specifically where to build these temple rooms and what the energy capacity would do for the planet.

The Hall of Water also contains an actual time travel device that only the highest initiates talk about and use. I remained in awe without words except my internal chant.

I ventured into the Hall of the Earth and sat on the floor in all its cold dampness to take in the energy of the Solstice and mind-blowing art. I allowed the sacred art and symbols to enter my whole being to activate dormant parts of myself.

The Hall of the Earth is dedicated to the male principle to the Earth as an element, planet, and to the memory of past reincarnations. It is a circular-based room, which develops into a cone shape toward the ceiling. Four doors fashioned in Tiffany technique with colored glass represent the sun, moon, earth, and the people. They open onto stairways, altars, and corridors leading to other halls. Behind two portals dedicated to the people and the moon, there are three windows in Tiffany glass, whose centers represent the elements of the zone in which they are found (water, earth, and fire). The outer parts represent a prayer linked to the search for spirituality. The walls recount the story of humankind according to Damanhurian philosophy.

I did not run into Peter much; this was definitely a solo experience. The next hall to explore was the Hall of Metals. This hall represents the different ages of humankind. According to Damanhurian philosophy every age is linked to a metal or element. The eight windows located in the walls read like a book. Information on the metal as an element, its atomic number, atomic mass, fusion temperature, dilation co-efficient, chemical notation, Latin name, and its correspondence in the tarot can all be read in the window. A landscape forms a background to the face concomitant with the age represented in the window. The flower of Damanhur, the dandelion, is depicted in its various stages of growth, from bud to full flowering. In this hall the story of humanity is told about the contrast between negative aspects (represented by the vices) and positive aspects; i.e., whoever defends the fire of awareness. The vices of humankind are expressed in the floor mosaics; the six human figures represent pride, egoism, pessimism, falsity, lack of awareness, and self-destruction: the images are immersed in a sea of dark stone. The ceiling depicts the positive part of the battle. Five warriors with conventional weapons (bow, sword, and lance) and spiritual weapons (a magical instrument and a book containing knowledge) oppose the vices. The figures move in a clockwise direction in relation to the floor.

Next stop, the Hall of Spheres to sit and dissolve into a colored sphere. This hall is four by seven meters wide. The ceiling and top of the walls are covered in 24-carat gold leaf: this material was chosen because the gold functions as an insulator. Eight crystal spheres are displayed in eight niches decorated with mosaics, as another sphere is displayed inside an aperture in the exposed rock at the central point of a wall. This hall is positioned at the exact intersection point of three important synchronic lines. From here it is possible to contact all points of the planet and transmit messages, ideas, and dreams to help create harmony between co-existing nations and stimulate the development of "peoples." Between one sphere and another there are sculptures in reconstituted stone, which provide support for the various chalices: the sculptures represent the union of the masculine and feminine principle, which creates energy and power.

I had a funny experience in this hall. I sat on a cushion facing a clear white sphere and began using one of my other mind busying mantras; *I am one with God.* I was repeating this over and over again in my head as usual. One of the men from our retreat group, Bud, sat down next to me and all of a sudden my mantra changed to, *I am one with Bud.* I must have repeated it several times before I noticed what I was doing. I started chuckling to myself and decided to keep repeating, *I am one with Bud.* I thought this must be appropriate since it was so spontaneous and why not? It did not matter that I did not know this man in the least, hadn't even spoken to him, and he even seemed a little standoffish. Maybe just disoriented, who knows? Of course, *I am one with Bud!*

The last hall I meandered my way into was the Labyrinth. Written descriptions cannot convey the magnificence and magnitude of this place. Experiencing it firsthand in the physical, knowing I was opening myself to the encoding symbols, was all I could convey.

The Labyrinth is currently in the form of three high naves with pointed arches connected to one another by three further naves, to create a labyrinth, with many possible pathways. This hall is dedicated to the story of humanity, which is related through the representation of divine forces that have been worshipped on the planet throughout the centuries. This artistic work unites different cultures and peoples. The Divinities are depicted in sixteen windows using Tiffany technique combined with cold-painted glass.

I found my way back to the Hall of Mirrors so I could rest next to Peter; no sleeping, just rest. I had no idea of the time and what was next, but what seemed like a couple of hours later Orangutan quietly directed us to stand up. We stood facing each other as he suggested we greet and hug everyone. I found myself being drawn to Bud even though he was not inviting me to come toward him. I gave him a big hug and said,

"We did it!"

He embraced me openly at that point.

IT'S NOT WEIRD ANYMORE

We were led out of the temple and to a vehicle to take us back down the mountain to the visitor's center where our comfortable beds were waiting. I think we slept a couple of hours, ate breakfast, and went to the meeting room for a gathering of all the Solstice Temple participants. Just about everyone who spent the night in the temple gathered together in this meeting room for sharing. Each person expressed their experience, some profound and some funny. I told the crowd I could not believe that after lying on the thin mat I was not sore in the least. Bud shared the most thought-provoking insight. He said he had wanted to leave the temple for six hours while he battled his demons and dark thoughts. After the sixth-hour mark he felt calm and easily stayed put. It seemed the sixth hour mark was around the time I was next to him silently chanting *I am one with Bud*. I thanked Bud for taking on the dark for the others in the temple and maybe the whole planet for that matter.

Peter and I went back to bed for a while, got cleaned up, and joined the Damanhurian community outdoor stone circle Solstice ritual ceremony. This was within easy walking distance just behind the visitor center where we were staying. We joined the large outer circle of about 300 people. The sacred dancers were dancing; the ritual performers wore red and white robes and spoke Italian in front of a burning caldron. I had no idea what they were saying so I danced to the live drums in my small space in the outer circle and felt complete. Movement is my way of absorbing and sending energy, and words are not necessary.

The next day we took a magickal sculpting class. The teacher, Lamb, gave us our instructions with his heartfelt spiritual guidance. He instructed the new students to dance around the room and freeze in power poses, and had us pick one that we felt would be appropriate to sculpt ourselves naked in. He gave the old students a different assignment. He told them that 20 years ago Falco told the community that the chalice would take on a different form than the cup. Lamb asked the old students, and Peter was among them, to sculpt their impression of what form it might take. He showed us the selfic device he placed near us in the room to magnify our artistic abilities. The new students sat at a long, well-used conference table with a large hunk of clay at each chair. The old students sat at a different conference table directly behind me.

Lamb helped us get started with his gentle directions while our hands began to form the clay. If our figure appeared too small Lamb would come around and add more hunks of clay from our own pile that was given to us for the project. He showed us tricks for making our figures taller if they seemed too short. Only one out of eight in our new group had any sculpting experience. We were hypnotized and possessed as our hands moved the clay. I was so engrossed in what I was doing that every once in a while I would think, *Where is Peter?* I could not feel him in the room even though he was right behind me. Peter was just as focused and engrossed in his project as I was and could not be disturbed.

My naked figure was standing upright with arms and hands crossed over my heart. I started from the bottom up and created my foundation. I molded myself propped up against a lotus petal that I leaned my voluptuous round butt on. I wanted to form my hips and torso as honestly as I could. I think I ended up a little too short though. My favorite thing was taking tiny bits of clay to place as pubic hairs around my exposed yoni.

Lamb pried us away to take a lunch break. When we returned he asked us to switch projects and work on someone else's sculpture. We had to pause a moment and comprehend what he was requesting because we had grown pretty attached to ourselves. Once we sat in front of another's piece with their permission we dug in. One of the men at our table had not formed his genitals yet and the one sculptress in our group made a beautiful erect penis for him. He kept it with pride. I sculpted my favorite yoni onto the one in front of me and the woman did not keep my enhancements. After about an hour of fiddling with someone else, Lamb had us go back to ourselves again to finish up. I used the same technique for my head hair as I had for my pubic hair and was working on the details of my face when Lamb asked us to finish as much as we could in fifteen minutes. I didn't feel quite done, but it would have to do. He gave us a piece of paper with the Damanhurian sacred language symbols and invited us to carve them into our naked clay bodies. I did this with exuberance and reverence at the same time.

Everyone's piece was magnificent and had a radiant quality to them. Some were alien and elemental-looking. One was mermaid-ish, another was elfish, and another was a powerful Goddess, etc. Everyone kept asking me,

"Have you seen Peter's yet?" with a half smile, half smirk on their face.

Peter's was his interpretation of the newly formed chalice and consisted of a male and female with arms locked facing each other as their genitals were about to be penetrated. The male and female creatures had little wings, pointy ears, and smiles on their faces as they happily gazed into each other's eyes. They looked kind of alien, elfin, angelic, and sexy.

Lamb asked us to leave the room for a short period and wait for him to call us back in. When we entered the room he had us sit in a semicircle and placed one sculpture at a time on a pedestal facing us. He asked us to imagine that we did not know who made these sculptures and we were archeologists who had just dug these up and they were thousands of years old. Lamb asked us to look at the statue on the pedestal and each give our interpretation. This was amazing, and even though we did not know one another, the insights that everyone described were the essence of the person. I was blown away by how my clay sculpture described who I was to a stranger and some of us cried it was so powerful.

We did not take our figures back home. The tradition was to leave the sculptures in Damanhur and the community would move them periodically to different locations around the property. This way your energy was being more strongly influenced by the energy of Damanhur and vice versa.

That night Peter and I met with Pooka (magickal animal), our wedding minister, to make a date and place for the ceremony. We decided on July first the full moon in the open temple at 4 p.m. This was after our retreat finished and the first day of the Intentional Community Conference. Most of our group decided to stay for the conference and could attend our wedding. Pooka set up an appointment for Peter and me to meet with him and have a counseling session to discuss Damanhurian philosophy for marriage and give us our assignment before the wedding.

The next day after our sculpting experience we were invited to the tree house community of Damanhur. It was wonderful to be in the woods and climb around all these little hobbit houses and see how they lived and learn how they began their community. Just like the underground temples they started with practically nothing. They lived in camper trucks and gathered all the building materials for their tree houses from the area.

The main reason we were interested in visiting the tree house community was for the forest concerts that the trees and plants actually give. Peter told me about witnessing this when he visited Damanhur the first time. The plant or tree was hooked up to electrodes like a lie detector and synthesizer and would start making the synthesizer play music. Peter said he could not listen to it without waves of emotion and tears in his eyes. Our tree house guide, Squirrel, had a houseplant hooked up that had been playing musical notes all day. She took us deeper into the woods and hooked up a tree that had never played before so we could witness it for ourselves. We could tell the tree was experimenting in the beginning and became bolder as it got familiar with the synthesizer notes. Squirrel explained that some plants that have been playing and practicing for a while sound very sophisticated and some are natural virtuosos from the beginning, just like humans.

One woman in our group had lived and worked in Findhorn, Scotland, the famous garden that teaches how to work with the nature spirits in any garden and it is a living, breathing, wondrous, example. While we were listening to the tree play the synthesizer, she telepathically communicated to the tree to hit higher and higher notes and it did just that. I was advised to add skepticism here, but I personally have none on this particular subject because the intelligence of plants feels normal to me and not weird at all.

The story behind plants playing music with electronics in Damanhur was someone performed an experiment with plants recognizing people. Several plants were placed in a room as one person came in and destroyed one of them in front of the others. One of the plants was hooked up to electrodes and a graph and as soon as the person who destroyed one of their buddies walked in the room the plant's graph went wild. Everyone else who passed through the room did not provoke any graph activity. A police detective found out about this study and decided to try and solve a murder case doing the same experiment. There had been a murder in a room with a plant, so he hooked the plant up to the electrodes and graph without the suspects knowing. As they walked in the room the plant's graph started moving back and forth wildly when one suspect in particular walked by. The detective was able to dig deeper into the suspect's alibi and whereabouts and convict him.

A community member from Damanhur heard this story and decided to do some experiments of his own; hence the concerts. One of the other amazing things a plant was able to do was drive an electric cart around following its owner like a dog and move itself into a sunny area and park. In Damanhur everything is alive, has meaning, and is respected. Three people in our group bought the plant devices to take home and experiment with their own houseplants playing music.

Our group had some extra time in the late afternoon, so some of us climbed a hill between the open temple and the underground temple. There is a park at the top that a spiritual humanitarian businessman donated to the government with an ancient turret lookout tower standing on it. Six of us gathered in a circle and performed the Holy Grail Vortex Activation. I was happy to have found an ideal spot to do the activation, especially in close proximity to the largest concentration of synchronic lines.

The next day Crotalo personally requested to drive our group to Turin and take us to the Egyptian Museum, where 14 Sekhmets were displayed and still activated. As I mentioned in my trip to Egypt with Delilah, Sekhmet was the lion-headed Egyptian Goddess whose name translates as *She Who Is Powerful*. She is sometimes destructive but her main qualities are as healer, mother, and protector.

Here is a little background about my relationship with Sekhmet. She has been my teacher for years. She has many names; my personal favorite is *She Whose Opportunity Escapeth Her Not*. Around 1994 I received a shiatsu massage that incorporated hypnotherapy. In this session the massage therapist took me on a journey. He asked me to breathe deeply and with every breath visualize myself descending down stairs that led deep into the earth. His voice took me further down the steps until I reached a landing with a closed door. He asked me to open the door, walk in, and describe the room. I saw an audience sitting in front of a stage waiting for me to stand in front of the podium. I said it was not so much that they were waiting for what I would say, but what I was emanating, which was the feminine essence. The massage therapist asked who was sitting in front of me and I saw Sekhmet looking directly into my eyes,

"What does she have to tell you?" he asked.

"Remember who you are, remember who you are, remember who you are." Three times like that. Wow! That was powerful.

Soon after that session I bought a Sekhmet statue, made a waterfall, and placed her in it. One time a friend came by the house with her two-year-old. The little boy gathered fallen flowers from a bush out front and placed them in the fountain as an offering to Sekhmet. Then he took his formula or milk from his bottle and started pouring it in the waterfall to complete the offering. His mother started to stop him, but I saw what he was doing and let him finish. He was teaching me about puja, the offering to the Deities.

Sekhmet later became my main altarpiece outside the waterfall; she followed me everywhere. She blended nicely with the Egyptian basement-healing chamber Cynthia and I created. Later when it was necessary for me to consolidate my belongings and move in with a friend I put the statue of Sekhmet away. While I lived with my friend I began attending the Rocky Mountain Mystery School, receiving initiations and practicing the teachings. The school asked the students to do a ritual that would confirm our commitment to the light. This consisted of taking our most prized object, something we held dear, and destroy it. Sekhmet's statue was the one and only thing I could think of that matched this request. I brought her out of her safe place and put her on my altar for two days and nights and communicated to her about the ritual. She was honored to be the one and felt our bond became stronger after that.

I performed my regular rituals and took the statue of Sekhmet in the backyard, which went down into a ravine with blackberry bushes. I took my hammer, smashed her statue into tiny little pieces, and threw them down the ravine. My roommate and friends could sense her presence in the house even though they knew nothing about the ritual. They would make comments like I see or feel someone over there and I felt someone walk by me. Another friend said she could see an animal head like a horse or lion's head.

Crotalo drove our group in a van to the Turin Egyptian Museum and explained to us that the Sekhmet statues were still active. Her energy works like this: during the waning moon the statues will suck energy from you, and during the waxing moon the statues will send you energy. On the full moon, which is when we were there, it's an equal exchange of energy. Crotalo said to be discreet and touch the statues without getting caught. He would try and distract the guards so it would be easier for us to commune with Sekhmet. As soon as I walked into the room with all the Sekhmets I felt very energized, emotional, and tearful. Peter and I stayed in the room and breathed her in as we touched her discreetly and took blurry snapshots. Peter has an old relationship with Sekhmet too. Dan and Rio told us about previous excursions to this museum when some in their group fell to the floor convulsing while experiencing past-life recall.

There were many rooms and floors with lots of artifacts, mostly Egyptian. One room on another floor had the entire original Egyptian Book of the Dead on papyrus. I was unable to stand up on this floor and had to sit down and keep myself from falling asleep. I had no energy in front of the book and was fine in other parts of the museum. I went back to the room of Sekhmets and met up with Joanna, a woman from our group. I had not thought about my Sekhmet statue-destroying ritual until I was back in the room with Joanna. I explained it to her and she looked at me and said,

"You also embodied that ritual from your accident."

Oh my God! I had not put that together at all. I just stood there motionless, taking in her observation and allowing it to sink deep inside of me.

When we returned to Damanhur Peter and I met with Pooka for our marriage counseling session. He told us that Damanhurian marriages renew their vows every year. This does not mean we must come back to Italy every year to renew them. He asked us to separately write our intentions for the union and then come up with our vows. Pooka said that many couples have different reasons for marrying and some are shocked when they state their reasons separately. Pooka felt it was best to have a discussion with each other before the wedding and create vows from there.

The last time Peter was in Damanhur he had a Damanhurian wedding with his last relationship before me and Pooka was the minister. Pooka taunted and teased Peter by saying that Damanhurian marriages renew their vows with the same person, not marry a different person every year. I found this to be quite humorous. My understanding of Peter at the time was that he goes full bore into a relationship and desires the woman he is with to love him as deeply as he does her. Scorpios are intense and if you are not willing to go deep, you may push them away.

When Peter was in Damanhur the time before with his girlfriend, he told me about a selfic relationship bracelet he bought in the jewelry store. He said Falco's high priestess wife handed it to him with a look that Peter read as, *You are not going to like what this does at first, so good luck and God bless*. Peter said his relationship at that time began to fall apart despite his efforts to keep it together. He became very sarcastic about the bracelet and thought it was causing damage until he met me. Not until then did he believe the selfic bracelet actually worked and was working all along.

Peter and I began to work on our intentions for our relationship. I am so brief I came up with a couple of sentences and he came up with a long list. He gave much more detail and poetic beauty to our vows than I did, and I will tell you what they are later during the wedding.

Our room was at the end of the hall and kind of private and we made love every night. We were asked to move to accommodate new visitors to a different location down the hall and more in the middle of the hallway. It was so hot with no air-conditioning that the windows needed to be left open. I guess our love-making kept the women in the next room awake since the windows were open. They teased us in the morning and actually said they appreciated it and gave us compliments. A couple of days later we were asked to move across the road to the Atlantis House because a new bunch of tourists needed our room, which slept three. We were able to make love without disturbing anyone I hoped.

After we met with Pooka the open temple was having a concert, so we all walked up to the amphitheater to sit and wait for the musicians. I watched the people gather and looked to the right and below me and saw a familiar face. A friend from Seattle named Isis. I raced down too greet her.

"Wow! What are you doing here?" I exclaimed.

She was just as surprised and excited as I was. She knew about my accident and had not seen me until now and was amazed at how I looked. Isis and her boyfriend were traveling all over and were on their way to Turkey. They had visited the underground temple tour earlier in the day and were very impressed. Isis' boyfriend is an artist and one of his sculptures was on exhibit in Florence, Italy, and since they were so close they came to visit Damanhur. I invited them to our wedding. Isis really wanted to come, but was depending on a host couple to drive them around and they were staying in Turin with their hosts. She would see what she could do, but they would definitely be back for the *Full Moon Oracle* event.

The day after the museum trip our group hung around the visitor center and made appointments for healing sessions. Peter had a massage session with Seahorse, an amazing healer who uses the selfic technology in her treatments. All of the selfic devices tap into the motherboard/mothership of the technology; a humongous piece of equipment, with many large copper coils and large and small alchemical spheres weaved together. Peter loves Seahorse's work and has experienced her treatments every one of his visits to Damanhur. I chose to try the yearly maintenance selfic chamber and thought it might help heal my head injury. I am always open to new healing experiences and will try different methods when I trust the people behind them. I entered a very dark room and was directed to lie on a hard white medical bed (very Star Treky) and waited for Dr. McCoy. While I lay there, Antelope lowered a large selfic device from the ceiling to scan my body. It hung about six inches above me and slowly moved up and down my body, stopping in areas that needed more attention I suppose. It was a 15-minute treatment and it supposedly lasted for a year. When I was finished I left the room to join the others as they waited their turn for whatever session they requested. I noticed I had not felt any different immediately following the treatment and had a lively discussion with my group for an hour. Then I began to feel funny and could not follow a conversation nor participate in one. I looked at Peter and said,

"I feel like I am tripping, I need to go to our room and rest."

We walked across the road and field and made our way to the Atlantis House and crashed in our room for three hours. Wow, what a session! I have no idea what it actually did; I just trust the Damanhurians and try new methods periodically so it's hard to know what specific benefit I gained from each one. These healing sessions marked the last day of our retreat.

The next day we said good-bye to two in our troop, and the rest stayed for the Intentional Community Conference and the wedding. Peter and I attended the morning talks before the wedding at 4 p.m. The best class was with Dr. Rima Laibow and her husband, General Bert. They happened to be in Rome for a Health Freedom conference and one of the speakers from the Intentional Community Conference asked them to join him in Damanhur. I was particularly pleased because I had been following the doctor on the Internet and the desperately needed service she and her husband provide. Did you know that our health rights are being railroaded if we don't take a stand? The pharmaceutical drug cartels are discouraged that people can heal themselves and stay healthy with natural remedies and a healthy diet. I am sure it puts a hole in their pocketbook and it appears they think they own all the money. Dr Laibow and Gen. Bert have been traveling from country to country educating governments singlehandedly about CODEX

Alimentarius. CODEX's sponsors are big Pharma, big Medica, big Chema, big Agribiz and big Biotechna and our health rights stand in the way of their agenda. Dr. Laibow said the way to fight them is with real science. She said there are companies that are paid to write bogus scientific reports to back the BIG's products. Dr. Laibow said the way to fight back is to back up our position with factual science because the fake science does not hold water when compared to authentic science, every time. When her talk was over I approached to hug and thank her and ended up crying in her arms, overcome by gratefulness for her work. I regained my composure and invited her and Bert to our afternoon wedding and she thought she might adjust her schedule to attend. To learn more about CODEX, check out the resource section in the back of this book.

We happened to run into the couple we took the *Erotic Massage* class with in Harbin Hot Springs, California at this event and invited them for a quick lunch. They were happy to acknowledge that they followed through on their word about meeting us in Damanhur. We invited them to the wedding, but they had other plans and said they would meet us that night for the monthly *Full Moon Oracle* event in the open temple amphitheater.

Peter and I needed to skedaddle and start preparing ourselves for the big wedding, even though it was pouring cats and dogs. It had not rained much the whole time until now and I knew it would clear up for the wedding. Joanna from my retreat troop gave me a massage, fixed my hair, and anointed me with frankincense and joy essential oils. I loved having my body prepared like this. Joanna and I worked a little trade and I gave her a 22-Strand DNA Activation in exchange for the massage and she threw the hair treatment in as a gift. She and I connected like sisters; we seemed very similar in our thinking as healers.

Around 3:45 p.m. our group began the slight uphill climb behind the visitor center to the open temple. The open temple does not have a roof and means it is open to everyone, including the weather. Sure enough the rain stopped just in time. The floor in the open temple is terra-cotta color and made of stone with sacred geometric designs. The spot Peter and I picked to stand was at the top of the apex of the pyramid with a circle around the point. Just past this point was a closed iron gate that leads to the amphitheater with a large stage and altar with a gigantic quartz crystal in the middle of the stage. The open temple is lined with tall Greek terra-cotta columns and statues of Medusa, Pan, and a few others of which I was unsure of their identity.

What was left of our retreat troop, the Damanhurian newspaper reporters, Seahorse, and of course Pooka, gathered round for the ceremony. Peter and I kept our Mexican wedding rings, which Francisco, our timeshare guru, jokingly married us with, and used them for the ceremony. As soon as I anointed Peter with frankincense and joy oil blend, Pooka started the wedding service. I was unsure if he was speaking straight Italian or the Damanhurian sacred language; all I know is I had no idea what he was saying. Pooka gestured for us to say our vows, so we read them together to the small gathering and here they are:

Laura & Peter
Two are One

1. *We intend and choose to see the divine in each other.*

2. *We intend and choose to see the blessings of our past relationships and not give characteristics and habits of those in our past to each other in the present.*

3. *We intend and choose to be a complement to each other and not a completion.*

4. *We intend and choose to be committed to working through hot button issues and use them as a way to grow.*

5. *We intend and choose to be more aligned every day in that which is unconditional love.*

6. *We intend and choose to be a beacon to others, that they are nourished by the spiritual, mental, emotional, and sexual harmony that this love that we share is creating.*

7. *We intend and choose for this relationship in love to be a portal for the divine unseen to enter into the material and experience itself as ecstasy.*

8. *We intend and choose to constantly expand our truth into the unknown, embracing Sacred Love without fear.*

9. *We intend and choose to use each other's strengths to more fully engage in life.*

10. *We intend and choose to start our day together with this prayer, Mother/ Father God, we offer ourselves as pure conduits for Love, Light, and Abundance to flow into this realm. We give thanks and adoration that you are in this life through us, by us, with us, and as us to ever better know ourselves together more perfectly this day and forever more.*

LAURA LEGERE

Amen and Blessed Be,

Con Voy (Italian for "We are with you")

The group appeared deeply moved by our vows and requested copies. Pooka gave another gesture to place the rings on our fingers and I guess he pronounced us husband and wife and had us sign some papers. I did not have a bouquet to throw because the Damanhurians do not cut flowers for the purpose of a dying decoration. Joanna gave me her hat to throw and I cannot remember who caught it. Champagne was uncorked, poured, drank, hugs were given, pictures were taken, and the rain held back long enough. It started to pour buckets again as we finished up. On several occasions I have experienced at the end of an intensive retreat the rain coming down in waterfall proportions. I view this as a spiritual cleansing in recognition for the work people have done for they're clearing and forward progress.

The *Full Moon Oracle* was next on the agenda that night and once again I knew the rain would let up. It poured and poured and poured, and everyone was wondering whether they would attend because it was so wet. My thought was, *Even if it's raining hard I will be there. This was a rare opportunity and I am, "She Whose Opportunity Escapeth Her Not."* Around 7 p.m. people began to gather in line for the amphitheater and the rain lightened up and quit as I expected.

The *Full Moon Oracle* is a monthly event held; you guessed it, on the full moon. Anyone can request an answer to his or her question from the Oracle as long as the question is more internal than outward. For example, asking when and who your next romantic relationship will be was not acceptable. The better question would be: What might be hindering me from attracting a partner? These questions must be emailed a month or two in advance for preparation.

Soon the crowd made their way to the stone seats looking down at the stage. Peter and I were married on the other side of the stage just a few hours earlier and the *Full Moon Oracle* event felt like a continuation of our ceremony. We found seats in the middle and looked for Isis, her boyfriend, and the erotic massage couple from California. They were easy to spot and it was just as easy to move around and visit. It was a beautiful scene looking from a high point in the stone bleachers straight past the lighted crystal on stage and the rows of terra-cotta columns with lit torches as dusk was emerging. The ritual began with African drumming and kept building from there. The sacred dancers hypnotized us with their undulating movements and hand arm mudras as they embodied the drum rhythms. I was unable to stay still as usual and remained seated, dancing with my upper body on the marble seat while I watched the ritual unfold. There was a huge burning cauldron on stage with four High Priestesses dressed in long dark blue robes wearing tall silver pointed hats. I believe the main thing the Priestesses were doing was privately giving Oracle answers to the individuals who asked ahead of time while they stirred the ritual fire. These were personal and not necessary to share with the hypnotized crowd that was having they're own experience. The dancing and drumming kept taking the crowd deeper and I got swept into the ritual and could no longer sit and dance. I left Peter and joined some others up toward the top of the bleachers, let myself go, and danced my butt off. That is how I absorb rituals with music; I must dance through it to grasp the nonverbal information and cleansing. The trance continued for two hours and the clouds parted, night fell, and the full moon began to peek over the horizon directly dead center between the temple columns. We were in awe of this particular moon because it was a terra-cotta-colored moon that matched the temple floor, the columns, the torches, and the lit quartz crystal on stage. The image is burned in my mind forever since we were not allowed to take pictures during the ritual. What a wedding day!

The next day was filled with speakers from different communities all over the world, but mostly from the United States. I became very bored with so many speakers who were not very prepared on top of having monotone voices. Peter and I decided to skip some of the talks, relax, and take some walks and a nap.

A woman in our group requested a meeting with Falco in the evening and Peter and I made sure we were around for that. Falco had very little time to spare, so this was another rare opportunity. The woman was starting a community in Ashville, North Carolina and wanted Falco's advice. She explained the extent of what she had in progress already. A rich couple who bought property were developing lots for hopefully likeminded neighbors. Falco asked if the properties were for individuals and the answer was yes. He expressed to her that she only had a village and not a community. Falco told her when it is left up to the individual you will have chaos because they can sell to whomever they want and you have no control over the new property owner's intentions. He said the key of the foundation for any successful intentional community is a core group of people who agree to dream the same dream. Then they all invest their money together in the property and cannot withdraw as agreed upon and when others want to join the same agreement applies. Falco started with 15 people and created an amazingly successful community that has a 32-year track record and growing. He gave us one whole hour of his time, all the while ignoring his pesky cell phone. What a gift! Damanhur has a constitution that is easily accessible in their bookstore and consists of 20 simple principles that might assist anyone considering creating an intentional community. In my view many good-intentioned people come up with the money first, start the project, and hope likeminded people will join them. It may appear that way in the beginning, but because the foundation was not laid out, it more than likely would fall apart as I have witnessed a few times myself.

On our last night we went to a small Italian town with our group and a few Damanhurians to have a beautiful last supper. Pooka picked us up at five sharp the next morning, drove us to the Turin airport, and sent us on our way. I had arrived in Italy without being able to see my ankles and left wondering whether I would ever see them again since they had eluded me the whole trip. Sitting for almost two days on a plane was too much for my lymph system. By the time we arrived in

Seattle I had clubfeet and could barely fit into my sandals. My sister Ruth picked us up and dumped us off in a daze and we crashed for a long lost slumber.

~ 26 ~

After recovering from jetlag I decided it was time to start bringing things back into my life that were put on hold while I recovered from my accident and fell in love. Okay, so what was I doing before Peter? The main thing was my PGP. I began to fit it back into my schedule and felt it would be particularly useful in my relationship with him, and believe me, it definitely was. To put it mildly, Peter assisted me in finding my negative triggers that being single does not illustrate as readily. One of the triggers I remember was Peter's tone of voice sounding cutting and condescending and I would express anger because in my perception it felt like he was calling me stupid. Proving I was not stupid was one of my core issues I foundn in PGP and a theme with several friendships I have had. I let Peter know he was helping me find my crap to work out with my PGP coach. I would apologize for being a queen "B" if I flew off the handle and thank him for showing me my issue. He said he had never experienced anything like it in any relationship and has quite enjoyed the journey. The other benefit of PGP is when Peter was angry I didn't take it personally most of the time. As I mentioned before at this point in our relationship, stuff was getting handled and cleared so fast I couldn't remember the specific issues and the PGP would say that means the issue is gone.

Soon I was fitted with braces to repair my bite by Dr. Geoff Greenlee at the University of Washington. Boy! I forgot what braces were like. I had braces for two years when I was a teenager, not expecting to ever wear them again. I had one more year to go it seems. My gums got extremely sore from Dr. Geoff's wire twisting and precision care. I looked forward to having my bite back, closing the gap between my teeth, and getting my health back on track. Dr. Geoff did a great job making sure my bite lined up as well as being available if I had any problems.

It felt so good to be back in PGP, getting reacquainted with my friends in the program and taking a spot in Goals Lab. Goals Lab helps everyone reach their goals according to their interests. Each person has an infinity goal and works on 90-day goals that build toward the infinity goal. Goals Lab model works in 90-day increments with weekly goals that build toward the 90-day goal. The 90-day goal builds toward a one-year and five-year goal and so on. I worked on my business all last year and came out way ahead. This year I decided I would challenge myself and do something I have never done before and write a book. I believe I would not be this far along if not for the lab and all the support.

In the meantime Peter would like to generate more income and take a part-time job. He is an avid practiced organic gardener of 25 years, so my friend Kitty the acupuncturist suggested working for Full Circle Farm selling organic produce

IT'S NOT WEIRD ANYMORE

at the local farmers markets. Peter and I got online, pulled up Full Circle Farm's website, created a resume, and emailed it late one night in July. The next morning the farm called, asked for an interview, and put him to work selling their produce at four different farmers markets around Seattle; some part-time job! He worked four 10-, 11-, 12-hour days and loved it because he loves the product, talking and watching people and getting to know the area in a hurry with all the driving around. We ate the best just-harvested vegetables. Peter doesn't let me cook much because he is a grill man and I am not a grill woman. He grills outside just about every night all year long and grills or steams his farmer's market veggies. It's an easy sell to his customers because he can tell them an easy way to cook the produce and how good it tastes. I also think his deep, sexy voice with his gentle southern accent and his good looks (tall, dark, and handsome) is a draw for his customers as well.

Peter has another talent that is delightful, entertaining, and worth mentioning. He knows all the classic rock artists, a bit about their personal lives, quotes them, and can do impersonations. He owns a large music collection and speaks about music better than any DJ I have ever listened to. His knowledge and taste in music extends beyond classic rock and is versed in R & B, jazz, country, and classical. I had envisioned him having his own radio show soon. With his gifted bird calling I never get tired of listening to him make whatever sound he feels like expressing in the moment, oh and those delicious succulent spiritual poems he writes are an added bonus. I think they would make wonderful, uplifting song lyrics to raise consciousness.

Here is another sampling of his poems:

Swirling Mass of Love

Swirling mass of all truths, physical and unseen, the divine paradox

See how it is all interwoven

Each piece nourishing the other

The example for living in joy, ecstasy and abundance is all around us

Now the hour arises when we stop acting like we cannot see the truth and

largeness of our divine selves

Where we are ever free to enlarge on ways where we can serve and adore the

divine in each other

To delight in our differentness and yet as one

LAURA LEGERE

All accepting the divine paradox into our hearts

From there all things come into realization of love

Never wavering from its desire to ever more perfectly see itself

Swirling but still

Masculine and Feminine

Darkness and light

Ascending and Descending

All things and nothing

Beginning and end and neither

By Peter Walker

Not too long after our dynamic trip from Damanhur, another important event date was on the horizon. July 17th 2007 was an event called *Fire the Grid*. One woman prepared and communicated this date around the world for years. She said her angel guides suggested this was hers along with earth's destiny to have people around the world focus positive energy at the same time on this date. *Fire the Grid* was one among many such dates and they all carry a particular energy frequency that benefits the planet.

Pacific Standard Time for this event was 4- 5 a.m. and it was recommended to choose something you felt would send positive energy through the grid. Dance is my way of sending the most powerful frequency of ecstatic energy. Peter and I woke up at the designated time and danced naked to Peter's music picks with appropriate lyrics to match. After this kind of joy, ecstasy, and foreplay for 45 minutes, we made mad, passionate love and fell into a delicious dreamy slumber. We felt we had accomplished our assignment and conveyed our message, "Make love not war."

Now we seemed to be settled in with Peter working, making his own mark, and my massage healing practice moving full steam ahead, and PGP helping me with the book.

~ 27 ~

Peter continued his detox program and experienced extreme itching for quite some time. This is what happens when the body wants to eliminate toxins by pulling them out through the skin. It can show up like a skin rash or just itch. At times he felt like tearing his skin off and kept making himself bleed in places. He had tried all kinds of natural anti-itching creams; they helped some, but there were nights he could not sleep from the scratching. My health education told me it was better to detox now and get it out of his system than have him age a sick old man with dementia never knowing what happened.

Continuing with the subject of health, nutrition, and detox, PGP sponsored a Medical Intuitive instructor, Caroline Sutherland, to teach her truth about health in the individual. I opted to attend because Caroline seemed to have another health piece of the puzzle for me. After indulging in Italy I was looking for a kick-start to get me back on track. Caroline gave each student a health evaluation sheet and a quick two-minute intuitive reading on their level of health. Then she expanded on the major health issues and myths in class. This was where I learned about wheat, dairy, and caffeine in more detail than I had known before. The combination of caffeine and dairy can block the lymph system. Wheat is an inflammatory food and can cause sluggish lymph and arthritis. This explains why I did not see my ankles in Italy, after sitting in planes and airports for over 36 hours and eating homegrown organic wheat, dairy, and coffee, no wonder my body protested.

Caroline had worked in an Environmental Medical Clinic, where patients were tested for food allergies and chemical sensitivities. She tested thousands of patients and came upon interesting health data that she shared in her classes. After testing so many patients she noticed she intuitively knew what someone needed to eliminate or add to their diet and lifestyle. The simplest way to convey this is:

The 8 Components to Peak Health, Longevity, And Weight Reduction:

1. Eliminating Allergic Foods
2. Candida Yeast Elimination
3. Low Carbohydrate Intake
4. 10 or more glasses of water a day
5. Organic Food-Based Personal Care Products
6. Hormone Balancing
7. Moderate Exercise
8. Healthy Emotions

Caroline said in her experience most everyone across the board were allergic to wheat, dairy, soy, and sugar. Corn and citrus were somewhat less, but not far behind. Coffee would be healthy to let go of as well. I did not eat hardly any dairy before my Italian excess, so it was easy for me to return to no dairy. I don't have a problem with corn on the cob except it got caught in my braces and became a pain in the teeth to eat. Caroline's recommendation for me was to stay away from wheat, dairy, soy, sugar, lower my carb intake, eat more animal protein, and balance my hormones.

LAURA LEGERE

Note: As of today 4/21/10 my intuition no longer desires animal products. I receive protein through greens, nuts, etc.

Did you know the leading cause of death in the United States is Western medicine and our diet? It's called SAD, the Standard American Diet. One of my teachers told me an experience he had while on a plane during the Thanksgiving and Christmas holidays several years ago. He was sitting next to a man who said,
"This time of year is very good for my business."
My teacher asked,
"What do you do?"
He replied that he owned a funeral home and that people literally eat themselves to death this time of year. He added that he was absolutely forbidden to write articles about it.

Of course I brought my new knowledge home to Peter and he rejected it in the beginning, as usual. Once I showed him what was more beneficial for us to eat, instead of what not to eat, he started shopping differently and even cooking the new way. Butter is the only dairy that is good for you; thank Goddess! We replaced wheat bread with 100% rye bread located in the refrigerated section of the health food store or co-op. Peter loves his dairy so I introduced him to goat milk and goat cheese. He no longer woke up in the morning full of the mucus that cow's milk can cause. I got him on wheat-free cereal and waffles and he can absorb way more carbs than I can and stay slim. For a sweetener he uses agave or maple syrup, much better than white sugar. For a fun dessert we have pure coconut ice cream on occasion. The main part of our diet consists of animal protein and lots of local organic veggies. We had become quite creative, substituting ground nuts with shredded coconut for wheat to batter fish, oysters, and chicken and whatever else we could think of that it would work with.

I was using rice milk for my smoothies and found it contains carrageenan, a commonly used food additive that is extracted from red seaweed by using powerful alkali solvents. These solvents can remove the tissues and skin from your hands as readily as would any acid. Carrageenan is in soy, almond, and hazelnut milks as well. I found hemp milk to be the safest of the non-dairy milks, since it does not contain carrageenan and all other ingredients are organic.

Up-date: Since this writing the makers of hemp milk have added carrageenan and the organic rice milk has removed it, so I am back to rice milk. It is so important to keep reading ingredients.

Balancing hormones is the longest task when you are over 50, in peri-menopause, and recovering from a head injury that really messed up my thyroid. Not to mention Peter's age and all his health issues messing with his hormones. Caroline suggested Bioidentical Hormone balancing, which is using natural substances that match your own hormones. Big Pharma hates this and their chemical hormone replacement has lost business due to their extreme side effects. They have tried to squash the Bioidenticals and have not been successful, but they keep everyone on they're toes because they continue to try.

Wifey suggested that Peter and I find a Wiley Protocol Bioidentical Hormone Naturopath. T.S. Wiley has trained and certified MDs and NDs with her hormone protocol and wrote a book about the mainstream medical deception and remedy called *Sex, Lies and Menopause.* Suzanne Somers interviewed T.S. Wiley in her book *Ageless* and suggested that balancing hormones can be a way to prolong youth. I went to T.S. Wiley's website and found the closest certified Bioidentical Hormone ND in Kirkland, Washington. Dr. Lucinda Messer was booked a month in advance, so we could not see her until mid September.

Watching Peter suffer from detoxing and itching was not easy, but I felt confident we were on the right track with a wellspring of support and resources to back us up. Peter and I traveled well together and continued with our travel plans through his healing process.

~ 28 ~

Our next travel adventure that I had planned a year ago (meaning before Peter was in the picture) was Washington, DC for the Young Living Essential Oil Convention the beginning of September. Since we would be so close we made the trip home to Roanoke and Lynchburg, Virginia, to visit our parents and introduce ourselves. We left Labor Day weekend and drove to Portland, where our flight took off. Peter used his timeshare points for the tickets and the closest flights available were out of Portland. I had friends, Sue and Michael in Portland, and they were so hospitable; they took us to the airport after spending a whole day and two nights with them.

Just before we flew east we heard that there were two class-four hurricanes headed toward Cozumel. A friend informed me that residents were fearful and getting prepared for the worst as before. I said my prayers and rituals and waited to hear some news since this was the closest test to see if the Holy Grail Vortex Activation Peter and I set really worked. The first one was Hurricane Dean and seemed to dissipate and lose momentum as it headed to Cozumel, then veered south and hit land. The next one behaved the same way and left property and people intact. Well, who knows? I'm just glad everyone was safe.

We arrived in DC in the afternoon before rush hour, rented a car, and drove south as fast as we could to beat the rush. Peter and I realized we had overestimated our arrival date by a day. We had a mix-up in communication about the convention dates and he made plane reservations ahead of the event. DC is very expensive to stay overnight and we were booked in a hotel for the convention for an already expensive stay. Our best budget option was drive four hours to Lynchburg,

Virginia, and stay with Peter's old friends Jeffy and Donna. It was strange for me to be thirty miles from Roanoke and not call or see my mom for another five days. We spent the night and had planned on spending the day with Jeffy and Donna, but realized that the registration and a welcome dinner for the convention was that night. We left in the morning and drove four hours back to DC. The rental car that we were not going to use for four days needed a reservation as well and added to the most expensive Young Living Convention I have ever attended in.

Washington DC had a very dark energy feel to it and the convention was not cost effective for Young Living or the attendees. I received an intuitive hit that the cost was irrelevant to the service the Young Living healers brought to the area because it was the anniversary of the 2001 September 11th twin tower bombings. Peter and I had plans to gather some friends to perform the much needed Holy Grail Vortex Activation at the Washington Monument.

This was a significant trip because I would see several concerned people who were on the Young Living cruise with me and were anxious to know how I was doing. After the convention I would visit my family and friends in Roanoke who had been a tremendous support and had not seen my new face yet.

It was fun running into familiar people, especially the cruise people. They were so glad to see how good my progress was coming along and that I was very much alive. I received much more attention than I was accustomed to. I bumped into Mary Hardy and had a brief conversation with her. There were about 4,000 people at the event, so it was a miracle to run into people I knew. I reminded Mary Hardy who I was while she gave me a big hug. I said,

"The crash happened because I needed to stay and finish doing the vortex activation work at the ruins."

"I knew that, we'll talk," she said.

I did not see her again. There was the husband, wife, and son team Wifey and I always ran into at Young Living Events. They helped Wifey marathon pack our suitcases on the cruise ship so she could depart with all our belongings. They were particularly glad to see me. The husband said he thought I was gone for good because the description sounded so bad. The friends Peter and I hung around the most were our aromatherapy teachers, Sheila, Gary (husband and wife team) and Tammy. Peter was taking their class when he got the call that I had an accident. They helped Peter through the traumatic news, taught him how to care for me, and gave him some much needed, hard-to-come-by essential oils to bring me in Cozumel.

Sheila and Gary are from Alaska and have become good friends of ours. I would like to share a mind-altering tidbit about them. Gary grew up with several McDonald's fast food restaurants as the family business, and as a result Gary and Sheila owned three McDonalds, became wealthy workaholics, all the while raising kids. They were monetarily rich, unhappy campers. In 1997 Gary began reading Neal Walsh's *Conversations With God* books and had a major epiphany.

"You mean I don't have to live like this?"

IT'S NOT WEIRD ANYMORE

They sold their business in Anchorage, Alaska, and moved to the middle of nowhere, Tok, Alaska. The only concerns they had were making sure their kids caught the bus to school and back. While the kids were away at school Gary and Sheila made love for hours until the darlings came home. Now they have many imaginative venues, too many to list here, for creating wealth that reflects their essence. They're *Heart Institute* is listed in the resource section. Okay, back to the convention.

Some friends from my hometown of Roanoke were at the convention as well; the husband and wife team, Kimball and Anne Egge, with Kimball's sister, Merry, and mother, Doris. Peter was no stranger and reminded Kimball where they had met in Roanoke on a mutual friend's front porch. What a kick Doris was and she also happened to be a good friend of my mom's, beginning in the *League of Women Voter* days. This was the first time I met her and it was a pleasure spending a little quality time with Doris and her family.

I found out later that Doris had an amazing accident story of her own while in Athens, Greece. She's a very petite 84-year-old and was hit by a car at age 82 as she was crossing the street while trying to keep up with the hurried tour guide. A female motorist was in a hurry as well, struck Doris, and she flipped over the hood and landed in the street in front of the car. They initially thought she must be dead and were quite surprised when she stirred a little. The woman driver was devastated and extremely distraught since it is a major offence to hit a pedestrian. The Greeks have really cracked down on their crazy driving in the last few years. As Doris lay in the street a policeman leaned down over her body and informed her he would throw the book at the motorist. He would put the motorist in jail for months until a trial; she would lose her job, be away from her husband and kids, and basically ruin her life. Doris being the gentle soul she was would have nothing to do with ruining someone's life. The ambulance came to transport her to the hospital and the woman motorist accompanied her. She became quite an asset and could speak English to help Doris communicate with the doctors. The main issue facing Doris was a broken left femur bone that needed surgery. The Greek motorist came to the hospital every day and brought Doris food and water because Greek hospitals do not provide these items. The patients' families supply all the necessities. The motorist felt indebted to Doris for preserving her life and Doris was glad to have assistance with the language barrier, food, and water. The motorist diligently cared for her until Doris' daughter and son-in-law arrived and even then it was difficult for the motorist to leave her bedside. Doris' hospital stay amounted to three weeks and surgery for a cost of $3,000, much less expensive than my Mexican adventure.

Doris attributes her recovery to Young Living Essential Oils and the NingXia Red high antioxidant juice Young Living makes. She walks slower and has pain in her hips still, but is progressively getting better and has a great attitude. You would never know by being in her presence that she was in pain or had an accident. She has a very youthful, humorous charisma and is not one to choose mental suffering.

Peter reminded Kimball that they have mutual friends in North Carolina, Dan and Rio Watson, our Damanhurian retreat facilitators. I was still amazed at how easily Peter integrated into my life and became immediate friends with my friends and had familiar connections already. So many people would hug him for the first time and say things like,

"You are my hero," and, "Thank you for taking such good care of Laura." They were sincerely appreciative.

Peter and I knew who to invite for the Holy Grail Vortex Activation at the Washington Monument. Wifey was not as available since she had several of her business associate trainees to attend to. Sheila, Gary, Tammy and another friend of theirs, Monica, walked with us to the monument. We got as close to the structure as was comfortable in the grass. I handed out the ritual and said a prayer calling in all our guides, guardians, angels, and masters. It seemed as if we were invisible to the tourists. When we finished, we were surrounded with birds in all the different configured rotating circles created by the ritual. It was an extraordinary sight to look upon. Sheila broke the silence with,

"Masters dismiss," and that instant every one of the birds flew away.
The ritual felt incredibly powerful with more company and the main purpose for coming to DC.

Our group wandered over to the Lincoln Memorial and paid our respects. As I stood standing in front of Abe, I started laughing to myself because I was reminded of the movie *Thank You for Smoking*. In the movie the main character, a smoking lobbyist, was kidnapped by anti-smoking protesters, drugged, and left naked in Lincoln's lap with nicotine patches all over his body. He was taken to the hospital and woke up to a doctor telling him he was lucky because his smoking saved his life, but he could not smoke ever again or he would die. I regained my composure and began to read Abe's wisdom on the walls. I felt as if I was standing in front of a master who may even have participated in our ritual across the lawn.

The convention was winding down and soon it was time for us to head south to visit our parents. We drove to Lynchburg to visit Peter's mom and dad, Geraldine and Irvin, at their assisted living complex. Geraldine, or Geri, had some neurological damage from four back surgeries and was in a wheelchair; however, she can drive that thing like nobody's business. Irvin had his health issues and in spite of this he got around just fine. I enjoyed them both. We stayed for dinner with Peter's sister Debbie, her husband, Gary, their daughter, her daughter's husband, and they're four small children. Debbie brought her mother-in-law and a feast for dinner to the assisted living complex for everyone. Her grandkids kept us occupied, entertained, and busy until they wore us out and it was time for them to go home and go to bed.

Geri and Irvin's assisted living complex offered Peter and I our own suite to spend the night. It was ten times more luxurious than the DC hotel, plus it was free. We made love as usual and had a late morning rendezvous with Geri and Irvin to say good-bye for now. We were off to Roanoke 30 miles away to visit my mom, Liz.

~ 29 ~

My mom is a very interesting character and one of my best friends. She helped me tremendously with finances when I was in the hospital and was gradually letting me pay her back. She was very grateful to Wifey and Peter for staying with me in Mexico. At that time my brother made a nice gesture and offered to bring Mom with him to Mexico to take care of me. I said it was not necessary because Peter, my new love would do it. My thought was, *This would be too many people and way too expensive because three people cannot stay in my room*. Peter was completely a new concept to them since I had not been in a relationship for quite some time. Needless to say, Mom was excited to finally meet him in person.

Mom, Liz, has been a community activist most of her life. Her main profession was a social worker as the Housing Authority's Director of Social Services Apartment Management. Among her many projects for the community, she brought Planned Parenthood to Roanoke and was acting president for several years. At the time of this writing she still volunteered as a counselor at the clinic. She is a member of the Sister Cities program and as a result has had many interesting foreign guests stay in her lovely large brick gumwood colonial home. She loves company and on occasion rents rooms or just has visitors. Liz is a dynamic, youthful, artistic musician, 82 going on 62. She is a jazz pianist and still has her own gigs. All her body parts are still intact; she doesn't take medications and for the most part is not in any pain. It took years for her to let me carry her luggage at the airport. I think she's finally okay with it now. She's lovely, fun, humorous and likes her martini. Liz would say her health and longevity secret is M & M's (music and martinis). I hope she doesn't mind my description here. Love you, Mom!

I will never forget my trip to Greece with Mom the spring of 1997. I was 41, the youngest of our tourist group; everyone else was 70 and over. We teased the heck out of each other in front of our tour guide and the group. Mom kept telling everyone I was a great belly dancer and of course I was expected to entertain. I would tell everyone she was a great jazz pianist and she would cower and get embarrassed because she was expected to entertain as well.

The night I was not expecting to perform I became very sick with a terrible cold. As I entered the restaurant there was live Middle Eastern music playing and our guide picked me up and plopped me on top of a table to dance. I felt like death warmed over, but no one knew. I danced my jig and was off the table in no time. I received many compliments and requests for belly dance lessons. Okay, it's Mom's turn now. A few nights later our guide set Mom up to play with a Turkish violinist and they were magnificent together. Liz really surprised herself, but I always knew she could play without her sheet music.

Toward the end of our trip Mom and I stayed up late one night drinking in the hotel bar with one of the men from our group. He turned us on to a drink called Bloody Brains. I think it was vodka, cream, and grenadine. Man! It was strong and tasted pretty good. I don't remember how many I had, but I'm sure it was too many. Mom and I decided to call it a night because we were indulgently sauced. We could barely find our way and it was a wonder that we didn't fall down the long flight of marble steps to our room laughing and stumbling and finally landing in bed. We rolled around on the bed giggling like college girls and passed out cold. The next morning Mom was up early to have breakfast with everyone, but I was so hung-over I didn't make it to breakfast. She came back to the room and said everyone asked where I was. She told them we were out late drinking and that I just can't party like she could.

Liz was married to my dad, Bob, for 38 years until he died in 1994 of cancer. He was a community activist as well and stayed on the board of Planned Parenthood while selling Travelers Insurance. When I was a kid Dad played right along with my sister, brother and me as if he was our age. I remember we had a really hard downpour one hot summer and the rain was rushing high on the street curbs. My sister, brother, and I ran out and lay down in the street next to the curb to bathe in the rushing water and Dad came out to join in. The image of my dad lying in the street with rainwater rushing over him is burned in my mind forever. He looked completely content and happy. He gave lectures to men's groups about supporting women's health, had a wonderful sense of humor, and loved his golf. Dad was the life of the party and loved striking up conversations with strangers. While he was alive he was great at telling dirty jokes and appreciated that I enjoyed listening and laughing at them and whenever I hear one I can feel Dad around me. It's funny how Mom never really got his jokes, but after his death she started telling them as naturally as he did.

Let's get back on track and visit Liz.

~ 30 ~

Mom greeted Peter and me as the charming host that she is and was looking so forward to having us all to herself. Peter and Mom harmonized well together since they both are great humorists and had bantered back and forth over the phone for months. Mom's main planned events for us were a jazz night out down the street, a few meals with relatives, and a *Love Party* for Peter and me. We would figure out what to do the rest of the time in Roanoke.

IT'S NOT WEIRD ANYMORE

It was a thrill to be in Roanoke with Peter because this was very familiar territory to him as well. We drove around as if we had been together for years in this town and reminisced about this place and that place. We found we even had the same Blockbuster video membership, which was still current.

We performed the vortex activation in Mom's backyard; this seemed a likely place since we had done one behind our house in Seattle. The main beneficial power point in Roanoke was Mill Mountain at the neon star that overlooks and guards the Roanoke Valley. It is part of the beautiful, breathtaking Blue Ridge Parkway and hosts a Theater Play House and zoo. Peter and I drove up the zigzag road, parked near the star, stood underneath it, and carried out the ritual. Then we stood on the lookout deck and took in the grand view of the whole entire Roanoke Valley and Star City below. It was so lush and green that we could not see the houses below in the city; it was a beautiful sight to view and observe. We remained quiet and still and breathed it all in.

Peter met my brother David, his wife, Barbara, two of their kids, Austin, 19 and Hanna, 18. Their oldest, Jessie, 26, was living out of the state and could not be with us. Peter was welcomed as if he had been with my family all along. We shared meals with relatives who were very supportive mentally and financially with my recovery and wanted to see for themselves how I turned out. I was happy to see and thank them in person. My Aunt Ann and Uncle Hue were a delight to visit as well as Aunt Jane and Uncle Bill. Peter and I agreed that all the conversations were very thought provoking, stimulating, and mind-opening. Everyone seemed to have grown more conscious and awake as time passed. Pretty cool considering this was the Bible Belt and Peter and I had our assumptions about that.

Peter made his famous crab cakes for Mom one night. We bought 28 tiny blue crabs and spent four hours shelling. I will not do that again. Two Dungeness crabs in Seattle will make the same amount and are still quite laborious.

The *Love Party* was the main event for me because Mom invited several of my friends as well as hers. Most of the people who attended had sent their financial support and prayers for my recovery. It was great to see everyone and they were glad to connect with me face to face. Mom had a chocolate love cake made that read *Peter & Laura in Love*. Pictures were taken of us cutting and feeding it to each other and Mom said,

"The pictures prove you are married now," with a giggle.

I felt comforted that Peter fit right in with my family and everyone was appreciative of his gallant effort to help me recover from my accident from the beginning. I was happy that we came full circle to meet and thank everyone in person for they're effort as well.

The day after our *Love Party*, Peter and I began the drive back to DC to catch our plane and stop by Lynchburg to see Geri and Irvin one more time. Virginia is so beautiful with the bluish rolling hills, lots of farms, and ancient rural towns.

"I feel as if we were here in a past life together as Native Americans," I mentioned to Peter.

Something feels very familiar being together in this place with him.

~ 31 ~

It felt good to be back in Seattle and resume our routine. Peter admitted he felt a little homesick while we were away. I loved hearing that from him, especially since he was so new to Seattle.

He began selling his precious organic produce again. Not long after, he moved some produce boxes around the barn and hit his left shoulder on a nail. This began to itch more and became sore along with his other itchy spots. When I looked at it initially it looked like all the other places on his skin. Two weeks went by and he showed it to me again and it was swollen, red, raw, and oozing. I applied the oils because I thought we might be fighting the flesh-eating virus, not that I know what it looks like. It did not appear to help and I became very concerned and worried about him. I drove home from my PGP late one Saturday night thinking that I must check on Peter. When I arrived, he was sound asleep and expecting to get up early and go to work in the morning. I woke him up to check on his arm and shoulder; it looked worse.

"Let's go to the hospital," I said gently.

"No, I'll be alright, I am going to work in the morning," he said.

I got on the phone, called Wifey, and described it all to her.

"This is one of those times when you need to go to the hospital," she said.

She encouraged me to be a lot firmer with him and pressure him into agreeing to go to the emergency room. She also mentioned that her intuition told her that they might find something else.

I marched back into the bedroom and told him his condition could not wait and we needed to go now. He finally agreed and helped me pack a few things and got in the car at midnight. I decided we would go to Haborview Hospital, the trauma center for the Pacific Northwest. When I worked for the power company we were directed to ask to be taken to Harborview no matter where we were in case the other hospitals near by didn't have the staff or facilities. This came about from an experience I had on the job with an injured coworker. Since then Harborview had been the only hospital in my mind.

Peter was taken into the emergency room and placed on a stretcher right away. Wow! What service. I became calmer and less worried once the hospital staff took over to find out what was going on with him.

An intern began evaluating the situation and a doctor used an ultrasound machine to check Peter's arm for pus pockets. The outside of his arm did not show pus, but was oozing a clear liquid that concerned us. He was in incredible pain while the doctor ran the ultrasound pad along his arm. The consensus was there weren't any infectious pockets. Thank God!

I asked the intern to tell Peter to quit smoking and he stood over Peter and said,

"Stop smoking."

He then put Peter on a nicotine patch to keep his cravings down. He also gave us a phone number for a free *Quit Now* service where you receive a coach and nicotine patches.

The medical staff elected the intern to take a blood draw to assess the problem. I stood on the opposite side of the stretcher while the intern began to draw blood from Peter's vein. The intern was not that great at finding the best place to stick the needle and seemed to be fishing around. Peter wanted to say something, but his eyes rolled back in his head, his mouth dropped open, and I could not see any more rise and fall of his chest. I looked at the intern.

"What is going on?" I asked, bewildered.

"I don't know," he replied and ran out of the room to fetch the emergency staff.

I thought, *I should pounce on Peter's chest and bring him back* and then thought, *I am in an emergency room and there are people here who will do that.* Before the staff entered the room Peter took an involuntary, awkward, deep breath, and came back into his body. He looked at me like, *Where am I and where did I go?* He told me he went through the tunnel and was enjoying where he was. He mentioned to the beings he encountered that he did not want to go back and they said,

"You have to go back."

No sooner had that been said and bam, he popped back in his body.

"Thanks a lot," I said.

The medical team hooked Peter up to a cardio machine and were stunned to see his heartbeat with a large gap between the beats. They asked him if he knew he had an irregular heartbeat.

"Not really," he said.

A doctor looked at me and said,

"We may have to put a pacemaker in him and we're admitting him to cardiology now!"

I remained surprisingly calm as my PGP inner counselor kicked in and reminded me that we were in the collecting data phase, no sense in panicking. Panicking in an emergency room serves no one, and being the healer I am, my healing presence and focus kicked in. The irregular heartbeat must be the other something the doctors would find that Wifey mentioned.

Peter was wheeled into an open emergency room and hooked up to a cardio machine to monitor his heartbeat for a few hours. The male nurse told us this would show if Peter's heart rate would return to normal or not. I asked the nurse to display Peter's blood readings on the computer. The nurse said all his numbers looked pretty good and it did not appear that he was fighting a virus. The only thing that looked abnormal was his liver and we already knew that, because of the Hep C virus. I was relieved to find out he did not have some other serious virus.

Peter explained to us that before he had Hep C he tried giving blood and would completely black out. The second time he gave blood the nurse said,

"Mr. Walker, please don't ever come back here again."
My thought: *So this is his normal response for a blood draw?*
I looked over at Peter lying in his hospital bed.

"Now the roles are reversed and you are in here instead of me; this is how our relationship began," I said.
He grinned in agreement.

We spent the time watching the entertaining emergency room patients. I think there might be a television series about the Harborview emergency room. If not, there should be. Harborview is the Pacific Northwest's Trauma Center and if you don't have insurance or money you go there. I witnessed a prisoner ankle-cuffed in the bed next to Peter as he was looked over by the doctors and nurses. Outside the room were several homeless patients, one with a net over his head so he wouldn't bite or spit on the staff. At times there were weird outbursts of unrecognizable gibberish. Soon the prisoner was replaced with a young man on mushrooms having a scary trip. He seemed to be able to answer questions coherently and his birthday was identical to Peter's. Peter gave a cheery shout for Scorpios across the room from behind his curtain.

The nursing staff was amazing in spite of all the craziness, being yelled and sworn at. Everyone was pleasant, helpful, and humorous no matter what. I called them angels. After a couple of hours Peter's heart returned to normal and the cardiologist told Peter that a minority of people have his reaction to blood draws. He said that it was rare, but not unusual and Peter did not need a pacemaker. One down and another to go! Yes! I am glad that this was the thing that Wifey was intuiting. I am also grateful for my PGP keeping me calm while I waited for all the data, instead of making it up and panicking about something that did not exist. Even if he did need a pacemaker there was still no reason to be upset. The problem would be resolved either way.

The doctors decided to admit Peter to ICU so they could give him IV anti-biotics and monitor his arm. Peter's bed was among many with only a curtain of separation. He sent me home to get some sleep since we were not in Mexico and there was not an empty bed next to him waiting for me to jump in.

I fell into our bed for an early morning slumber. After resting I collected Peter's clothes and several things for his entertainment as well as some decent nutrition. We all know what kind of foodless food the hospital feeds the patients.

Upon my return to ICU Peter said he did not sleep that well with all the noisy patients. He told me he was educating the doctors and nurses about nutrition, es-pecially high fructose corn syrup. That stuff is in everything they serve and is pure poison to the body. Peter suggested they buy produce from Full Circle Farm and the doctor said the staff would like it, but the patients would not. I wonder if the patients like the current food that is served. It is ironic that people are here to heal, but quite the opposite may be happening as far as the nutrition is concerned.

Peter refused to drink the pop and coffee, or eat desserts. I brought him some delicious Phi Plus (51 raw organic ingredients of veggies, fruits, nuts, flowers, oils, and soaked grains) from the Wholefood Farmacy to chew on. I also brought powered greens and NingXia Red juice from Young Living. NingXia Red is a wonderful very high antioxidant drink made from wolfberries that grow in NingXia, China. It is a great liver tonic to mix with enzyme nutrient-rich green powder. Peter's nutritional needs were taken care of, thank God!

His arm looked better, the redness was reduced, and the affected area appeared smaller. He kept entertained by the cheerful, humorous angel nurses who peered in and out from his curtained room. According to what the doctors told Peter, he might have a staph infection, although the tests did not show it. They wanted to keep him another night, so I went home to rest up and fetch him in the morning.

Peter called in the morning and said that the dermatologist wanted to see him and the staff wanted him to stay until the afternoon. He would call and let me know when he would be released. In the meantime he was a teaching tool for the doctors, nurses, and students. They quite enjoyed his wisdom.

It was late afternoon around 3 p.m. when I went back to the hospital. Peter was all showered with clean clothes and could not wait to leave. He said the dermatologist had no idea what his skin issue was and called Peter an anomaly. He was given antibiotic pills to take for two weeks along with a month's worth of nicotine patches. Peter said he might as well quit now. I was happy about that.

Peter told me about the patients on either side of him with a marvelous impersonation of a woman. He said an elderly woman to his right watched TV very late at night and laughed so loud with her deep, raspy voice and kept him and everyone else awake. The nurses continually asked her to keep quiet so people could sleep. While she watched her TV she would talk to it and say,

"I know that's right," as she belted out her noisy laugh.

The old man on the other side of Peter had dementia and internal bleeding and did not know where he was and kept pulling his IV out. This went on all night long. Peter was so happy to be out of there, although he found humor in the elderly woman and her TV.

Peter took the antibiotics for a week and felt so horrible on them he could not finish the next week's worth. I gave him oregano, thyme, and lemon essential oils in gel caps to take. These can be powerful natural antibiotics but they did not last long because Peter's digestion could not handle them. He couldn't rub the oils on his skin because he itched so much from detoxing. The nicotine patches made him feel awful as well, so he stopped and did not take up smoking again, at least at that point, and his arm still looked bad.

Thank God he had an appointment with the naturopath. Dr Messer took one look at his arm and said,

"You do not want to mess around with that."

She gave him a prescription for an antibiotic cream that worked. His skin began to look normal again. Dr. Messer had Peter take a blood test before his next appointment with her in six weeks.

He started to complain about a sharp, burning pain deep inside his right arm socket. I tried everything I knew to get rid of it and nothing seemed to work. What a journey this turned out to be.

Peter's will was incredible; he did not miss work except the one day he was in the hospital. The farmer's markets were winding down for the fall and winter and Full Circle Farm offered Peter the opportunity to drive a truck a couple days a week. He received a couple of weeks off between the markets as well as deliveries and used his downtime to recover from his ordeal. Soon he was back to delivering vegetable boxes and working the winter farmer's markets on the weekends.

~ 32 ~

The fall of 2007 consisted of my massage practice and acupuncture healing treatments. My home yoga practice became stagnant as I allowed myself to get so distracted at the house, and with Peter there it was even more so. He was in a groove working for Full Circle Farm and tolerated his body through it all.

Kitty's loving acupuncture treatments were no small affair. She singlehandedly put my face back together. Every Monday morning I drove to her place, gave her a massage, then we traded positions on the massage table and she worked her magick with the needles on my face. It has been miraculous; my right nostril lifted to match the left, and the right side of my face, which received the most impact, lifted as well. Kitty said the needles remind my face that it has not completed healing yet. If I did not apply the oils and receive these treatments the right side of my face would be droopy and assume it was finished healing.

I met a woman who told me her mom had a car accident and had severe facial injuries like mine. She said the injury was very similar to mine and her mom healed up with a drooping face on one side and a very large scar. She said she never regained the feeling back in her face and just lived with it for thirty years until her death. This was interesting data for me to contemplate.

I am so grateful for Kitty's friendship, healing skills, concern, and love. She looked down at my face to see what needed to go where and carefully positioned small short needles along my disappearing scars. She placed flesh-colored bandages over the short needles so I could leave them in overnight and pull them out in the morning. Kitty used the long needles as well to assist the systems of my body to become stronger and run more energy. Once again I was reminded of all the health issues I am preventing.

Kitty is also a very skilled yoga instructor and helped me stay in shape and alignment. Her yoga is great physical therapy. Her practice goes back almost 30 years and looks quite fine on her. She is one cute beauty, with her long natural red hair, deep blue eyes, attractive smile, a slight front tooth gap, and gorgeous yoga body. She's always giving me beauty tips and even dresses me at times. My face, health, and wardrobe were in great hands with my dear friend Kitty.

IT'S NOT WEIRD ANYMORE

~ 33 ~

Thanksgiving was around the corner and Peter's skin was itching more intensely and his right upper arm pain continued with no relief with whatever I tried. We were invited to have turkey with Micki, my brother-in-law's brother's ex-wife, and all my brother-in-law's family. I have happily attended many Thanksgivings in the company of this same family and Peter and I were looking forward to being with everyone, but while monitoring his arm and condition it looked less likely that we would make the family gathering. We were still hopeful and focused on making it anyway.

Peter insisted on working early Thanksgiving Day for more pay and planned to meet the family in the afternoon. When he arrived home I took one look at his arm, saw how much pain he was in, and said we were going to the hospital again. He begged and pleaded with me to go to the family gathering and we could go to the hospital after turkey dinner. There was no way I could muster up an appetite, relax, and have fun worried about his condition. This was way beyond my new medical intuitive skills that I learned from a recent workshop I took from Caroline Sutherland. I was unable to hear my guidance because my mind would not quiet down to listen, plus I did not want the responsibility of making the wrong decision for him. I felt we needed a professional opinion and we could go from there.

"Please don't take me to that hospital again, take me somewhere else," Peter requested.

I packed his belongings in case he was admitted and escorted him to the University of Washington Hospital emergency room. This hospital was similar to a fancy hotel compared to Harborview and just what Peter ordered. He was registered and taken right away since it was a ghost town in there. The staff evaluated Peter and we were able to give them more information this time. The doctor looked through Peter's supplements, asked us what laundry detergent and body lotion we used. Peter's rash seemed to follow the sleeves on his T-shirt and the doctor thought it might be laundry detergent. Peter's blood test showed good numbers according to the staff and indicated he was not fighting a virus other than Hep C.

While I sat in the waiting room I was able to calm my mind and tune into my intuition. I was shown a pod like an encapsulation of something lying dormant inside of Peter's body that had been activated to vacate. His liver and skin were working overtime to assist the substance to leave. I picked up that it was mostly mercury and petrochemicals. My conclusion was that Peter's skin was literally melting off of his arms as a result of a combination of mercury and petrochemicals pouring out of his skin from detoxing. His liver was so overworked and compromised from fighting Hep C, mercury, and petrochemicals that it had nowhere else to exit except through his skin. I was happy to know he did not have a horrible condition and was just detoxing too fast, causing a healing crisis. The doctor decided not to put him on antibiotics, but gave him something to help with sleep and sent us on our way.

LAURA LEGERE

We called my sister Ruth and found out it was too late for us to drive an hour to meet up with them for a Thanksgiving meal. Peter and I met Ruth, Mike, and the kids at their house and devoured our Thanksgiving meal there. What a day!

Balancing our hormones, Peter's detoxing, and all of my healing treatments took up most of our focus, as our aging bodies had become our lab experiment. Dr. Messer worked patiently with us, tweaking our supplements, thyroid, testosterone, progesterone, and estrogen. I always had a lively visit with Dr. Messer as we shared our knowledge and experience about health, the FDA, the AMA, and the pharmaceutical industry.

The FDA was calling all compounding pharmacies and telling them to stop compounding the bio-identical hormones and the pharmacies were not complying with the FDA's request since there was no law against it. Big pharma must be getting desperate since they have failed over and over again to pass a law prohibiting the bio hormones.

~ 34 ~

I must take a moment here to give tribute to Elizabeth Gilbert, the author of *Eat, Pray, Love*. Reading her book really inspired my own writing. It gave me the impulse to dig deeper and get more descriptive, and like mine, hers was a spiritual journey. She had a wonderful way of expressing herself with amazing humor and insightfulness, particularly during her amusing drama queen phase. I had a mystical experience while reading her book. She had recently arrived in Bali in her story and I soon fell off to sleep extremely hungry. I began to dream that Peter and I were in Bali on a spiritual retreat and the resort was beautiful, with Balinese architecture and decor. Peter looked handsome in his colorful clothes and motioned for me to follow him into the workshop room. I said I would be there shortly and began eating up all the hors d'oeuvres to quiet my appetite. I kept eating and eating and found a bowl of coconut cashew fish soup, snatched it away, and sat in a corner gobbling it up. Peter peered out from the class to look for me and asked what I was doing. I patted my stomach and said I was very full and we both laughed. I woke up to find my Balinese statue, which sits perched high above the day bed on a wall shelf, folded into the bed covers with me. How strange and mysterious, but then again it's not weird anymore.

~ 35 ~

Next on our event list was the *Winter Solstice Feast*. Peter would be with me this time to experience my favorite affair of the year. Last year in 2006 I knew he would be here for 2007 and most likely the ones to follow. It was time to consult Delilah on any projects she might have up her sleeve.

IT'S NOT WEIRD ANYMORE

Delilah's skilled teaching partner, Dahlia Moon, was leading an early evening candle dance performance as a Solstice opener. Delilah delegated her old students to make a dance stage art installation so her partner Eric's Middle Eastern band *House of Tarob* could play all night for the spontaneous spirit-inspired dancers. As usual the Fremont Arts community of hippie and pagan artists decorated a donated warehouse and turned it into a magnificent medieval palace in ten days.

I brought Peter with me to the warehouse so he could participate in the decorating and perceive how a community project felt. Working as an artistic team is the purpose of the whole initiative while you build a sense of a fun sharing community. I helped create the dance stage with Kristine Hamby's artistic direction and many other dancers' skillful hands. We glued silver sparkles onto tree branches, propped them up with plastic pipe, and wrapped them in tiny white lights and red poinsettia flowers. The trees lined the stage for the dancers and musicians, with large Goddess figures painted on canvas as a backdrop. We decorated two separate archways to enter the space as these led the solstice participant to the Turkish lounge, equipped with Turkish carpet and pillows. The lounge was a comfortable place to watch the performances, with a couch, floor pillows, and a couple of rows of folding chairs.

Peter and I helped staple evergreens to the candle chandeliers that hung from the ceiling to light the medieval feast. Headpiece-making day was one of the most pleasurable events during the preparation. My sister and niece, Ruth and Robin, helped make fun, decorative headpieces or festive crowns since they both wanted to be included in the celebration too. I loved watching the evolution of the mandala being painted on the floor and the whole site come together.

It was time to dress Peter up in his scrapped together pirate costume. He put on my green harem pants, gold lamé shirt, sequin-embroidered vest with a large white lion on the back, swashbuckling blue- and gold-striped waist sash, and King Tut necklace. He was so entertaining to dress up; either that or I am a cheap date because I am so easy to amuse. This year seemed harder for me to come up with a costume. I didn't want to dress in a belly dance costume as usual and I didn't want to wear my gold lamé Goddess gown. I searched and searched the thrift stores for an outrageous ball gown that would fit me. I ended up settling for a sleek spaghetti strap velvet black dress that I could dress up a bit. I wore it with a heavy, weighted, short, multicolored sequined jacket. Something Elton John might wear. Okay, we were ready to go!

It was Friday night December 21st 2007 and Peter and I arrived early and waited in line for what seemed like an hour. We were entertained by all the brilliant, creative costumes along with our recognizable friends. The wait was due to the fire marshal's nitpicking. Every year some of the art installations have to be re-created last minute due to the fire marshal's orders. We were glad to have the added safety, but there are times when it's over the top and ego based.

Finally, it was time to enter with organic apple pies in hand for the potluck. We were welcomed by the greeting crew, who wished us a Happy Solstice and showed us the donation vase and we gladly chipped in. We then entered the headpiece room and searched for the perfect one. Peter selected a silver icicle-covered one with red poinsettias and I picked a dark red one with berries and red and silver streaming ribbon. Any one of these beauties would match my multicolored jacket.

Robin had a basketball game, so Ruth and she arrived a couple of hours later. They had other friends to meet as well, a mother/daughter team too. Next we visited with everyone, toasted, and waited for the bread breaking ceremony. I joined in to hold up one of the conference table-sized loaves of bread that passed over everyone's head. The main presenter blessed the bread and the singers broke out in song. Then everyone was asked to touch the closest person to him or her while the bread was broken and passed to everyone. This was the signal to begin piling up our plates and feasting on the delicious food that had been lovingly made for the occasion.

Dahlia Moon's students made their way to the mandala painted on the floor and gave a superb candle dance to *House of Tarob* on the main stage. Peter and I walked around inspecting the clever art installations and ran into Ruth and Robin just as they arrived. Their other friends had saved them a headpiece and it was a good thing because the headpiece room was picked clean. Ruth looked up at Peter's decorative crown a little puzzled and said,

"Hey, I made that one!"

Out of hundreds of these decorative beauties Peter picked Ruth's. Our life is amazingly synchronistic, isn't it?

The solstice ritual was very entertaining and hypnotizing. The last performance had so many different-looking characters in bizarre costumes doing weird things that I leaned over to Peter and said,

"This makes me think I'm tripping."

The Sun King effigy hanging over the ritual with everyone's scrolled prayers tied to it was lit and brought down with African drums in a fiery passion. The dance frenzy began and continued for hours while I danced with Peter, Delilah, Robin, Ruth, her friends, and a few others. The rest of the evening went too fast. I wanted to stay longer, but we were driving to Boise, Idaho in the morning to celebrate Christmas with Peter's brother Michael's family. Once again I was happy to welcome the sun's return on the longest night of the year.

We hit the bed by 1:30 a.m. and reluctantly awoke by 5:30 a.m., packed, and were on the road by 7. While we drove to Yakima I thought of the Stonehenge replica that I wanted to show Peter. I called my friend Ken to find out if we were going to drive close enough to visit the site. It would be an hour out of our way so we decided to make the detour and drive through the Yakima Indian Reservation. Washington's Stonehenge was built to scale on the Columbia River in Maryhill, Washington. It was built in the 1930s by Sam Hill a road builder, honoring some local soldiers.

I mistakenly left the Holy Grail Vortex Activation ritual at home. Stonehenge was a perfect place to perform the ritual and on the actual Solstice to boot. Peter and I decided to perform it anyway since the activation was part of us now. When we approached the structure there was no one in sight. I looked at Peter and said,

"Do you know how rare this is?"

We remembered as much of the ritual as we could and felt the intention was the most important aspect. Stonehenge sits on a beautiful piece of land just above the Columbia River Gorge and overlooks the vineyards that are scattered along the riverfront, a spectacular sight to see. The Holy Grail Vortex Activation on the Solstice at Stonehenge was a wonderful way to enter into the holidays with family and friends and set up a positive tone to proceed through.

~ 36 ~

Back on the road headed to Oregon on our way to Idaho. The weather changed as we approached the Blue Mountains and drove 200 miles in a snowstorm that worsened as we arrived in Boise. The eight hours it took Peter to drive to my house driving the same route and distance a year ago took us 16 hours to land in Nampa, Idaho. We drove an hour out of our way, stopped to investigate Stonehenge, pulled over to take a 15-minute nap that lasted an hour and a half, and drove in a snowstorm. The little extra slumber was understandable when you consider all of the gratifying deterrents except the snow.

I was welcomed into the family the same way Peter was accepted into mine. Peter's brother Michael, sister-in-law Sandy, and his niece Jackie were easy to converse with since they were informed about current events that the regular news does not convey; we had lots to talk about. The other aspect of feeling so comfortable around them was their spiritual nature. Sandy's mom was a well-known spiritualist and had an immensely positive influence on her family and community. I thoroughly enjoyed visiting and getting acquainted with this part of Peter.

They live on a beautiful nine-acre horse ranch with eight hunting dogs, twenty-three horses, and too many cats to count, and very different from Peter and my city life. Peter's brother Michael designed and contracted the construction of their gorgeous 3,500-square-foot ranch house. Michael and Sandy sold Pergo flooring at their floor-covering business and Sandy taught horseback riding as well. Michael had just received word that he had been hired as the regional Pergo rep and would be traveling to headquarters in Seattle quite a bit. Sandy's job would require more hours running the flooring business, and caring for horses is not a leisurely occupation either.

We arrived Saturday late and spent Sunday recuperating. Peter and Michael planned one of their favorite activities together on Monday, Christmas Eve, bird hunting with the dog pack. I decided to accompany them and take a walk in the mountains. Four of the dogs were in the truck bed, housed in their little dog kennels, and were aching to get out to run and point. The gentle rolling hills of the Owyhee Mountains were covered with short sagebrush, perfect for chukar birds to hide out. The dogs beat their tails against their kennels until they got free and were able to perform their natural instincts. A light sprinkling of snow covered everything and was easy to stroll through as the dogs ran up and down in a frenzied exercise to let off steam. I followed Peter and watched large jackrabbits hopping all over in the snow as they escaped the dogs and their disturbance.

We walked to the top of the first rise to get a good view; it all looked the same and appeared easy to get lost, even with a compass. After walking around for a couple of hours and no birds to speak of, we decided to head back. Michael kept calling for one of his dogs, Patch, because he had not seen him since he released him from the kennel. We called out, searched, and left Patch a kennel where the truck had been parked and covered it with sagebrush for warmth. We drove around the mountain searching and found dog tracks in the snow that led nowhere while the new falling snow covered more signs. The joyful day turned sad as we drove home with one less dog.

Michael said that eleven-year-old Patch had done this several times through the years and had always come back. That dog was a little crazy and could point and point and point even though he would be totally exhausted. Michael drove back to the sagebrush-covered kennel that night and returned alone.

Jackie, Peter's niece, liked to bake and made all kinds of pastries, cookies, pies, cinnamon rolls, etc. I did not have my regular food with me and decided to eat the festive food they had. I could feel my system getting clogged and knew I would clean myself out when I returned home, so I went with it.

Christmas day was fun as I gave everyone ionic footbaths that draw out toxins through the bottom of their feet. While Jackie's feet were soaking, she and I showed each other our conspiracy websites and conversed about all the unethical behavior in government. Peter's family was not big on wrapped presents, the same as my family, which made it very pleasant to relax and just be together as the gift, so offering a foot bath and intimate conversation worked well.

Christmas dinner was lovely, and we all felt fortunate to be in one another's presence. Sandy, Jackie and I created the feminine bond that I always welcome. Sandy said she was so glad Peter found me, especially since she had watched him go through all of his other relationships. She seemed to indicate that I was the best fit. What a high compliment!

Michael traveled twice on Christmas day to look for Patch and came back empty. The next day Peter and Michael looked again, talked to nearby farmers, posted notices about lost Patch, and notified the forest rangers. About six weeks later a local hunter found Patch's body curled up under a sage bush. He died doing what he loved and was probably so exhausted he crossed over in a peaceful sleep.

Peter and I said our farewells for now and headed for the road back to Seattle Wednesday morning. I was thankful for Peter's driving skills because we headed toward a more severe snowstorm over the Blue Mountains than the one we had arrived in. It looked treacherous as I reminded myself to keep breathing and was relieved I was not the one driving. Once out of the Blue Mountains the road was smooth sailing, dry and not much traffic. Then just 60 miles from home on Snoqualmie Pass the traffic and snow were abundant and slowed us down to barely a crawl. Earlier a tree had fallen over the highway and backed traffic up as if it were a parking lot. I kept track of our time and distance and noticed it took us an hour and a half to move five miles. We were stuck on the pass for about two hours when we finally broke through and flew home in record time.

We felt as if another milestone in our relationship had been passed, now that I had met the rest of his family and we had been together a full year. Peter's son Michael visited us a few times, traveling with his bands as a soundman with gigs in Seattle. His daughter Sarah was the only one left to meet, although I had spoken to her several times on the phone. She lives and works in Ohio and I looked forward to meeting her someday soon.

Peter and I had consciously participated in many specific spiritual events as well as created our own when called to and experienced intense health and healing crises so far. I looked forward to the day of Peter's complete health recovery and moving ahead without the busyness of doctors' appointments and downtime at home from feeling bad with low energy. Coming together with Peter has been the most intense beginning of a relationship I have ever experienced and has created a strong bond between us. I believe if we can survive a year like we just had, then we can survive anything and thank Goddess for our sound spiritual connection for helping us thrive through it all.

~ 37 ~

Once we felt settled back home after a couple of days we looked forward to the New Year. My next physical checkup was with Teresa and her biofeedback machine.

Teresa read my body and found my pelvis to be way out of alignment. I looked at Teresa and said,

"Sex."

"Bingo," she said and,

"Find a good chiropractor."

Thank goodness for Dr. Steve Polenz, a nearby chiropractor who uses a gentle treatment called *Koren Specific*. He took one look at Peter and me and said we seemed to be curved in opposite directions and laughed because he knew it was from sex.

Dr. Steve showed me how his gentle technique could help me with my head injury through regular visits for a short period of time. I have been amazed at how this gentle procedure put my pelvis back in place after the first visit and helped realign my spine so I could sleep on both sides at night. Regular visits have helped release the trauma stored in my head as well.

New Year's Eve was not near as eventful as the year before in White Rock, British Columbia, Canada, with the *Sex, Passion and Enlightenment* crowd. 2008 New Year's Eve Peter and I met our friends Kitty and Patricia and drove downtown to a party at a glass blowing shop. We didn't really know anyone, but they had great food, live music, and glass blowers entertained us performing their art. At midnight we went outside to stare at the Space Needle and watch the pyrotechnic display. A couple of puffs, then nothing for ten minutes and then another few puffs and nothing for five minutes and finally the show took off. It was normally a spectacular presentation and had been for 20 years, but this was such a dud. I heard that the TV and radio music that accompanied the fireworks ran out before the show took off. The news story stated that it was a computer glitch. Maybe this was a metaphor that 2008 would to be a very different year for the planet.

~ 38 ~

The anniversary of my accident was coming up on January 18th and what a year it had been. My sister Ruth remembered that day and called to wish me well and thanked me for staying alive. My friend Faye, the Cranial Sacral Therapist, and I began new cranial treatments on that day and Wifey called and asked if I was ready to go on another cruise because she won another trip with Young Living. She seemed hesitant at first and relaxed when I reminded her of our last words as she left the Mexican hospital.

"Let's do this again sometime," we chimed.

"I would love to go; I just won't ride any scooters."

"You bet you won't, and the events department was joking that you will have to sign some papers stating you will not do any scooter riding." Wifey laughed.

"Where are we going this time?" I asked.

Wifey said we would meet in San Juan, Puerto Rico, board the ship there, and cruise the Caribbean, St. Thomas, St. Maarten, Antigua, St. Lucia, Barbados. We agreed to meet April 8th in Puerto Rico three days early to take salsa lessons. *Yes, the start of this year was taking a different shape.*

Peter's health had improved according to our naturopath, Dr. Messer. A blood test the end of January showed his Hep C viral count had dropped significantly. He was still itching like crazy and had not physically felt energized, since the scratching kept him from getting proper sleep. The biofeedback machine showed mercury in every panel viewed, so he still had a way to go.

Two months went by and the biofeedback machine read Peter's stress level again. This time his stressors were way low and his itching had almost come to a halt. Teresa said she did not find any liver anomalies and his mercury level had dropped dramatically. The slowing of the itching could be that his liver was on the mend. I put him on a chelator tincture from Young Living called *chelex* that may have helped pull the heavy metals out of his body. I believe this tincture was what finally did the trick in conjunction with Dr. Messer's protocol. Peter drank gallons of NingXia Red high antioxidant juice from Young Living because it could assist his liver and may help lower his Hep C viral count along with the chelex. I could hardly wait to see his new blood test. I was very proud of Peter's persistence to keep up the protocol even though he felt miserable for over a year. It was all worth it I kept telling him!

Kitty gave Peter an acupuncture treatment and believed that his right arm might be out of its socket. She used tuning forks to re-set his arm and he finally felt some relief. Kitty is so talented. His arm may have been out of its socket since September 2007; if that was the case no wonder he had been in so much pain.

Next Peter had a four-hour session with Kristine, an angelic neighbor of ours. Kristine is a schoolteacher and works her magick on the side in her limited spare time. She read his tarot cards first and talked about how compatible he and I were for each other. She told him we had been together in several lifetimes and had played many different roles; for example we were sister and brother in one lifetime and mother and son in another. Kristine said that we had always had a very nurturing, harmonious relationship and this one was no different. She confirmed my take on Peter's body aches, pains, and itches, that his painful emotions stored for decades were on the surface and ready to be set free. Then she proceeded to work her angelic, magickal energies and reprogrammed his body to help release the old stuff.

Peter and I decided it was time to catch up with our *Contact Talk Radio* station friends, Cameron and Divindia. They invited us over for dinner so we could see the newer addition to their family, baby boy Phoenix. We have always had much to converse about with Cam and Divindia because we seemed to be on the same wavelength. I mentioned that Peter was looking into broadcasting school and would like to work for a radio station and Cameron said,

"I will teach you how to run the board."

We were a little surprised since we thought we were just going over for dinner. The evening took on a different turn and after two or three hours of discussion it was decided that Peter would have his own weekly hour music program and sell *Contact Talk Radio* commercials and host spots. How cool was that? Peter already had a radio name picked out, Peter Levon, the *Alternative Guru* Friday evenings from 5- 6 p.m. on 106.9FM-HD3 PST. Alternate cuts with alternate thoughts. We left their house excited about the new opportunity and venture.

~ 39 ~

Meanwhile the presidential election campaign was heating up and taking very different, unexpected twists and turns while Peter and I kept a close eye on the corporate media's propaganda spin. I have not mentioned anything about my political views except on big corporations infringing on our health rights, so I felt compelled to include my newfound political interest and participation in this chapter and in chronological order to the story. Up until this particular election I, along with many millions of Americans had not put much focus on politics because it appeared to be beyond our reach. I believe the Internet showed us that we might have an opportunity to have a voice. Americans could not believe how bad things could get and Bush's policies were a great motivator. I, along with many millions of Americans and countries around the world, took a new interest in who would become our next president. I believe the United States of America is actually the Corporate United States and is quite literally owned by corporations that do not have our best interest at heart.

In my opinion the campaign was so focused on terror in an attempt to keep us fearful so we would allow our rights to be legislated away. The Internet news and Comedy Central with Jon Stewart's *The Daily Show* and Stephen Colbert's *The Colbert Report* were the best sources of current events and the best way to make the news palatable. I believe they showed us what was real with such humor that you were not depressed while being informed.

I do not identify myself with any political party and would just like to vote for the best person, although the best person had not come forward to campaign for president in such a long time until now. I have read and listened to a Texas congressman for years and was convinced that he was totally one hundred percent incorruptible and could restore freedom, prosperity, and justice to our country. Along with Peter's support I became a committed Ron Paul Republican and declared myself a delegate at my precinct caucus. Ron Paul would bring the troops home immediately, repeal the Patriot Act, reinstate Habeas Corpus, get rid of the Federal Reserve and the IRS, create a sound money system backed by gold and silver, cut government spending and taxes, protect natural medicine, restore the Constitution, and more. He has been the one of the few lone voices speaking up for *We the People* in Congress since 1971. He voted against the Iraq war and consults the Constitution for all his decisions. He generated more money than any of the other candidates, none of which came from big corporations, just the citizenry. Every department in our military gave more money to his campaign than all the candidates combined. They want to come home and we want them to!

Ron Paul created a revolution by speaking the truth. The revolution is beyond the presidency while Ron Paul's *Liberty PAC* have run for office in every capacity and have designated themselves as Ron Paul Republicans. Whoever would be president was going to be held accountable like we had never seen before. All it took was for us to show up and learn as we go, like so many of us novices who had not been interested in participating until this election. As a delegate you could propose resolutions at the conventions. A new friend of mine, Al Shaefer, was running for Congress, was a Ron Paul delegate, and had several resolutions to propose. Rid ourselves of the Federal Reserve and the IRS, re-investigate 9-11, court accountability, etc. I proposed protection of natural health choices, repealing the Patriot Act, reinstating Habeas Corpus, making the president consult Congress for a majority vote for all proposals (especially war), legalizing hemp farming, allowing progressive science to proceed with free clean energy solutions, and releasing oil dependence. We could do this.

On Monday night March 24th, 2008 my district precinct caucus met to vote for delegates committed to attending the county, state, and national conventions. The Ron Paul Republicans in my precinct held a meeting the Friday night before to discuss strategies for getting elected. The good news was we did not have to declare a candidate preference. That would eliminate the tired old argument that a vote would be wasted on a Ron Paul delegate because he was not going to win and we want to pick a winner. The same horse race mentality that the *bought, paid, and sold their soul to the devil* media promotes.

The McCain camp was irritated with us once they voted for our group because they didn't know we were for Ron Paul. We had some interesting, lively exchanges as we mingled that night. How were we to effect change and bring in new ideas if we don't talk to one another, especially when we had very different perspectives? The precinct chair said this was the largest turnout in 20 years. I believe there were about 120 people compared to the usual 15.

Since Al and another man were running for Congress for our district, they were given ten minutes each to state their platform. Al's was humorous and heartfelt and the other guy said he was a reformed anti-war liberal Democrat and after 9/11 he became a pro-war Republican and was tired of all the lies about Americans losing their freedoms. The Ron Paul Republicans were appalled and thought the guy was mentally unstable. He may represent what was left of the old Republican guard; that's a scary thought and all the more reason to join the GOP and make changes on the inside. Anyway, that was my thought at the time.

Out of the 14-delegate allotment for our district we received seven and out of the 14 alternates we received nine. We stayed until it was finished and it dragged on for six and a half hours. Many people left and lost spots, but the majority of the Paul supporters remained and made sure we received as many positions as possible. At the very end Al's three resolution titles mentioned earlier were read and would be passed on for review. I finally placed my body horizontal at 1 a.m., but was so excited and wired I did not fall asleep for who knows how long and it didn't matter because I was extremely satisfied.

I have been reading several Internet posts on the Ron Paul delegate process across the country and the experience at my Republican caucus was not isolated. The same thing was happening all over the country. Yes, this was turning out to be a very different year indeed.

~ 40 ~

Wifey and I were looking forward to our next adventure together in the Caribbean and many wonderful events were taking place while we were cruising around. The Dalai Lama would be in Seattle teaching workshops for a week. Wifey helped put together an amazing healing event for Katrina refugees that took place while we were sunning ourselves in the Virgin Islands. Young Living donated lots of oils and massage therapists, yoga teachers, and counselors from all over the country converged in New Orleans to bring peace and comfort to the area. Oh, and Delilah was taking a large group to Egypt to dance, make music, and chant in the temples. I let her borrow my silver scarab bracelet and printed up a bunch of Holy Grail Vortex Activation rituals for her to use. April 2008 was a powerful month and particularly the week of the eighth through the sixteenth, our cruise dates.

Wifey and I called this the *cruise take two*. We had a most fascinating adventure ahead of us once again and greeted each other in baggage claim in San Juan, Puerto Rico. We had not seen each other since last September in Washington, DC at the Young Living Essential Oil Convention; she said I looked great, referring to my facial metamorphosis. We were both so happy to be together and knew we would have lots of fun dancing for three days prior to the cruise. Our cab took us directly to the charming Spanish villa, Wind Chimes Inn, in the ritzy part of town, where we slept, showered, cooked, slept, and slept some more.

The first night on Tuesday April 8th was too late to figure out where to dance and we found out that Puerto Ricans do not start dancing and drinking to live music until Thursday night and continue through Sunday. Wifey and I stayed in our room, visited and planned the next day. We bought groceries at the health food store because to our surprise we had a kitchen. Then we checked on a rental car to drive to the rain forest and found out where to salsa dance.

We slept in and got a late start on our day, and this same scenario would be repeated over and over again the whole trip. We decided to walk everywhere to get some exercise and this proved to be quite comical in some instances. We got directions to the health food store as it was a long way and we kept getting lost and would ask for more directions. One woman took pity on us and drove us to the health food store herself. Another woman in the store lived near our hotel and gave us a ride back. Wifey and I thought Puerto Ricans were awfully friendly and generous; we felt very welcomed, safe, and well cared for.

Now that we had enough food and water in our room, we could relax and plan our fun. The beach was a block away and we ventured there late one windy afternoon. We adopted the hotel cat named Elvis. Elvis had been living at the hotel for ten years and had a beautiful coat. Completely white body, black tail with a perfect white ring around the tip, black ears, black feet, and a few artistic black shapes around his head. He let us pet him while he guarded our door and eventually ventured into our room. The hotel clerk said Elvis had never let him touch his beautiful coat and said many guests were not allowed that privilege.

Our little outing for health food took up a good part of the day. We had time to fix a meal, watch *American Idol*, take showers, and get fancied up for our salsa dancing evening at the Marriott 12 blocks away. As soon as we arrived a skilled

IT'S NOT WEIRD ANYMORE

Puerto Rican male dancer asked me onto the dance floor. He was very patient and talked me through the steps with his calming words; soon I picked it up and was dancing like a professional. Once you understand the simple foot placement, you can move your upper body in many delicious ways. My belly dance skills have come in handy on numerous occasions and this was definitely one of them.

I looked around and found Wifey was with another very skilled salsa dancer. She was having a wonderful time being glided around the dance floor. After a while it was time for me to take a break and drink my wine. My dancing buddy became very persistent and kept asking me to dance constantly. It was a bit annoying and I was feeling claustrophobic. Toward the end of the evening he asked where I was staying.

"The cruise ship," I replied.

This would be true in a few days and kept him from pursuing me any further and he departed very disappointed.

Wifey was having a pleasant dance experience with her new friend; he gave her his phone number and said he would be at the Marriott the next night and would love it if she was at the hotel as well. We would think about that since there were other spots we wanted to check out. I think we hit the hay around 2 or 3 a.m. This proved to be the earliest bedtime for our Puerto Rican adventure.

We slept in again while the rain forest trip seemed to slip away on this day anyway. We walked to the open market, where Wifey heard that Friday nights all the market vendors close up shop, break out their instruments, play salsa music, and dance in the square. This was Thursday mid afternoon and kind of quiet. The only purchase was a delicious coconut, pineapple, banana drink for $1.50. Then we hailed a cab instead of walking back to our digs because Wifey was nursing a blister on her foot and experiencing quite a bit of pain.

Wifey cooked dinner while I read her the beginning of this book. After I read my account of immediately picking myself up off of the rock, walking out of the ditch, and assessing the damage. Wifey turned around and looked at me, excited and confused, and said,

"You need to change that, you never moved, you were lying in the ditch until the ambulance carried you out!"

"But that is distinctly how I remember it," I said.

"That was your light body walking around," she replied

"Did you ask me if I was okay and I answered you with a no?" I asked.

"Yes, that did happen," she said.

"I thought I answered you standing up. Wow! This adds a whole new dimension to the experience," I replied.

I began to contemplate what it felt like walking around in my light body and recalled it so vividly and very physically. It hit me how close to death I may have been and I remember feeling a bit defiant about it as well, hence the phrase death defying. Wifey said that I soaked two large beach towels from the cruise ship with blood and never needed a transfusion. Thank Goddess!

LAURA LEGERE

It was time to change the subject and return to our musical evening ahead. We took our time getting ready, watching TV and showering since the evening started around 10 or 11 p.m. We checked with our activities director hotel clerk, Jeannie, about where the best dancing and music venue would be this night. The Neorican Café in old San Juan was the place she suggested. We walked to the Marriott to check out the music there first. It was very crowded and the music did not appeal to us. We saw Wifey's dance partner from the night before from a distance on the crowded dance floor and decided to hail a cab and go to Old San Juan. I was happy about going to another venue because I did not want to encounter my dance partner from the previous night anyway.

The Neorican Café had an awesome salsa band with very few people in the place. Many people were standing outside talking; we found out later that this is their custom. No one was on the dance floor, so Wifey and I danced together and inspired other women to get up and move. There was one wild male dancer that motioned Wifey to dance. He was moving his body in some very interesting ways and every once in a while would nudge Wifey to turn. It became obvious he was only dancing with himself and wanted everyone to watch his crazy, unique, exclusive style. Wifey said he would turn his backside to her, place his butt in her hands, and belt out,

"Yeeeehaaa!"

He came back to our table, leaned over to Wifey, and said,

"It's just me, myself, and I."

Wifey looked at me and we both nodded in agreement.

It was fun to watch Puerto Ricans, male and female, dance together; they have amazing moves and showed so much joy dancing with each other.

The band took a break and Wifey and I ventured outside to talk to them. They were very young, about 21 and married with kids. One of them gave us his relationship philosophy, which went like this.

"Other women are like little snacks here and there with no serious feelings, but your wife, now she is like a full banquet that you are totally in love with."

We laughed and I mentioned that he could write a philosophical book about it.

The last set began at 2:15 a.m. and all of a sudden the dance floor and the café were packed. We closed the place down at 3 a.m. and hit the sheets at 4, slept till noon, and started our day again. The rain forest kept slipping farther and farther away from us.

We found a great hippie restaurant down the street called Pinky's with a yoga studio above and a Laundromat next door. It was time to do some laundry with all the sweaty dancing. Wifey was very familiar with Laundromats and saved my Victoria's Secret wireless bra from losing its shape in the dryer. It needed to air dry so I could wear it in the evening; therefore I hung it on the large straw hat I was wearing. After snacking at Pinky's and finishing our laundry, we walked down to the beach to check out a fancy restaurant. We wanted to have one night of fine dining before we boarded our ship. We walked in with our backpacks full of

clean laundry and checked out the menu. I looked at Wifey and said,
"I have a bra on my head."
Wifey replied,
"You have got to take that off right now."
It did not take long for us to decide not to eat there since Wifey is a vegetarian and could not find much to eat. We walked out laughing hysterically that we had walked into a ritzy place with a bra hanging from my hat.

It was time to prepare for our evening activities again and the aim was with dinner in mind. After showering, dressing up, and taking pictures of each other we proceeded to walk to a grouping of fancy eating establishments toward the Marriott. We ended up at a loud Mexican restaurant that had more veggie choices for Wifey and was not too terribly expensive. We ordered two large margaritas, listened to the customers sing Spanish songs, and had our pictures taken with two large sombrero hats while we sipped our drinks.

We walked down the street to see if we could hear our taste in live music to dance to. After walking, asking around, and not finding anything except the Marriott, we decided to take a cab to the famous Rumba Club. Our cabdriver was fun and talked us into going to another place called the San Juan Hotel. He assured Wifey that she would meet a hot Latin salsa dancer and we would not have to pay for drinks. The place was the most extravagant establishment I can ever remember entering. Marble floors, hardwood trim and ceiling, round marble drink bars scattered around, live band on a two-tiered stage high above the dance floor, semi-private rooms with silk curtains draped to the side, and the biggest chandelier I have ever laid eyes on. It must have been 50 feet in circumference.

Wifey and I were asked by a few men to stand at the bar and order drinks for us and them since they were not making any headway for their drink order from the bartender. We conversed with them while we radiated our feminine presence to hopefully get the bartender's attention. A jet-set Scottish businessman bought our drinks and his new male friends' drinks. Wifey looked at me and said,
"Are we supposed to hang out with him a bit since he bought us a drink?"
No sooner had she asked that when he gave us a cheer and walked away, never to be seen again. We looked at each other and said,
"I guess not. That was nice."
We made our way to the live music and looked for a place to park ourselves among the white couches and coffee tables facing the dance floor. Immediately a short gentleman asked me to dance. He was wonderful, very skilled and full of compliments for me, a complete gentleman and bought us drinks too. I danced with several men, all very different and fun. Wifey found her hot Latin dancer, James. They were lost in another world while he taught and glided her around the dance floor as if it were a beautiful poem. The same band played for six hours with only a couple of breaks, with three beautiful, petite women belting out song after song with so much energy!

Wifey, James, and I moved into the lobby while the band took a break and we could get some air. He was a lovely man who seemed to be awakening spiritually. Wifey was very turned on by that and I took pictures of them sitting in a big comfortable chair together and exchanging contact info. It was very early in the morning, the live music had stopped, and James offered to take us back to our hotel. We were appreciative and took him up on his offer. Our cabdriver was sure right on the money in his predictions; he was psychic or something, because it all came true; the salsa dancing men buying our drinks and Wifey's exclusive hot Latin dancer; another 4 a.m. night to remember. I don't believe the rain forest was in our grasp.

We had to be up early as checkout time was 11 a.m. and it took awhile for us to get ready. The hotel allowed us to leave our luggage in the lobby while we headed for Pinky's for breakfast, or more like brunch. We returned to lounge around on the furniture (lie horizontal on the couches) while I caught up on some much needed sleep and Wifey had essential oil business to attend to on her computer. We were required to board our ship no later than 6 p.m. and our sailing time was 10 p.m. Needless to say we had time to space out and be lazy.

I had an intuitive feeling that Wifey's and my dancing together has some sort of positive effect on the planet at strategic times. As I have mentioned before dance is my highest form of prayer and Wifey's added energy makes it much more potent. Wifey mentioned that her ashram called everyone to chant last night and she felt a little guilty for not doing it.

"Ah, but you danced all night with your hot spiritually awakening Latin salsa dancer, James. You were doing your part, don't worry," I said.

We caught a cab with all of our stuff and headed for the *Serenade of the Seas* Royal Caribbean ship around 5:30 p.m. We found our room, admired the balcony that Wifey insisted upon getting, and proceeded to Young Living's greeting party in one of the lounges. I was happy to keep sampling the high antioxidant NingXia Red juice and scored a full 32-ounce bottle for our room that would last the whole cruise for both of us. It was a wonderful energy boost after our energetic Puerto Rican dancing quest. It felt good for me to reintroduce myself to a few who were on the last cruise and wondered what had happened to me after my accident. They were so happy to see that I was doing quite well and that I came back for our *cruise take two*. Gary Young was unable to attend because he was critically needed for harvest in Ecuador, so he sent Mary, his wife, instead. She was especially glad to see me and to know that I was okay.

I was mainly looking for Mary Hardy in the lounge but ran into her on the stairs instead and reminded her who I was. We hugged and she said we would get together and carry out some activation work with new information.

Young Living had one of the many restaurants, Reflections, partially reserved every night for our group. Wifey and I ate there the first night so we could be with everyone, but Wifey's veggie, non-spicy diet did not agree with the fare there. We ate in the cafeteria from then on.

There was a show this night, but Wifey and I did not attend. We seemed to have gotten so engrossed in a conversation with our fellow essential oilers that we lost track of time. We went to bed early for us, around 1 a.m., and still managed to sleep in. We awoke in St Thomas, took a cab to a beach, laid around sunning ourselves, and swam in the crystal blue water.

Wifey was particularly looking for a newer acquaintance in her business, Londin. Londin brought her good friend Brent, and when we finally met up with them at the end of the first full day we stuck together like glue. We found we were in so much alignment with one another that it was uncanny.

Wifey had business associates to connect with while I attended the evening comedy show, which was quite good. I headed for the disco lounge to dance, opened the door, took one whiff of cigarettes, and left; it really stunk in there. I began to compare my last cruise on the *Grand Princess* of the Princess cruise line with this ship and found not all cruises are the same. The disco lounge on the *Grand Princess* allowed smoking, but their ventilation system kept the smell minimal. So much for thinking we would dance for a few hours every night before bed.

I must have hit the hay around midnight, woke up a little earlier, and Wifey and I made our way to the cafeteria. We met up with Londin and Brent for breakfast and had a lively conversation about our last cruise. One more joined our group, an old friend of Wifey's she met at an essential oil training years ago named Caleb. We filled them in about the Holy Grail Vortex Activation and as synchronicity would have it Mary Hardy showed up to fill us in on the latest. Brief introductions were given and Mary told us what was going down and asked if Londin, Brent, and Caleb were interested in joining the Grail Activation ritual at night on the upper deck. Of course they were, Wifey and I had just prepped them. Mary proceeded to tell us, according to the alternative Internet news, about a recent incident on April 2nd where Dick Cheney ordered a B-1 Lancer supersonic strategic nuclear bomber based out of Ellsworth Air Force Base to bomb Iran's Bushehr nuclear plant. According to uncensored Internet news, Russian military analysis, and the *Rapid City Journal,* Defense Secretary Robert Gates ordered the B-1 to change its course or be shot down. The US Air Force commanders launched fighter jets into the air against their own Naval forces and a F-16's cannon fire hit the B-1. The B-1 changed course for an emergency landing, the four-crew members were safely evacuated, and the plane was destroyed on the runway at Al Udeid Air Base.

The work Mary has done with the Holy Grail Vortex Activation was to help change the chaos our current administration was attempting to create. Many believe as I do that the current administrations plans were to start world war three so they could stay in office, declare martial law, and not have to resign. Mary believed by performing the activation with as many people as possible and focusing our energies for peace and prayers for the military to make peaceful decisions, we could turn it all around and actually manifest true peaceful relations with all countries.

LAURA LEGERE

Mary said she would be at the Solarium pool on deck 11 every night at 10 p.m. for anyone who would like to join the Holy Grail Vortex Activation ritual. I brought many printed copies of the activation to hand out as well. The added focus was to set an intention of peace over the Middle East by sending love through the Holy Grail Vortex to the Silk Road leyline and to the consciousness of the world leaders to perform, with free will, their duties with love, instead of terror. We appealed to them to act with the consciousness of the Christ energy. The Silk Road leyline was being set aflame with destruction and our intentional focus was to transmute these flames through the emerald light of love with the purpose of prevention and service.

The next morning our little breakfast vortex gathering seemed to be lost in a time warp, so when we decided to leave and get out and about it was almost noon in St. Maarten. We took a cab driven by *Joseph the Coat of many Colors* to a beautiful tourist beach with crystal blue water and pristine white sand that happened to be a nude beach as well. I appeared to be protesting nakedness since I had burned my body the day before and had on a long-sleeve shirt and long pants. I was not too keen on exposing my body parts because of memories of my burned body not having a good time in that condition. Wifey, Londin, Brent, and Caleb all went swimming while I watched our stuff. We laid in the sun with varying clothing. Wifey covered much of her body with her clothes and exposed her breasts to rid herself of those pesky tan lines. I began taking pictures of our group, as we looked so comical. A man walked by with two women and I overheard him say to them,

"Nudity is so gross."

He was not referring to my Wifey since he had just walked past a whole slew of people and had not noticed us. I mentioned this to Wifey and we laughed.

"Boy! He was really exposing his own hang-ups. I would not want to be his spouse," I said.

After soaking up enough sun we decided to sit in the shade at a pirate restaurant under the palm trees and ordered drinks and a fruit plate. We got lost in our time warp again. Learning about Brent, Londin, and Caleb was fascinating. Brent had broken every bone in his body as a sports thrill seeker, and two years ago while riding a bike a drunken truck driver hit him. He split his face in half straight down the middle. His skin was peeled back toward his ears. If no one had seen it happen he would have bled to death. He remained unconscious for four days. His face looked perfectly normal now, which is a good omen for me. He and Londin met in a healing workshop seminar and have been friends ever since. Brent was very humble, a little mysterious, and has powerful healing abilities. I am unsure how he came into his healing skills, but my assumption was through the many times he may have faced death. He helps people rid their body of physical and emotional trauma, as he is a vehicle for higher spiritual energies to move through. This can be a description for many modalities, I suppose, but we all have our unique gifts.

Londin was a kick in the pants, a beautiful young woman on a mission to teach people about the oils and walk her talk as absolute health. She was a filmmaker, news reporter, and public speaker on a roll. Traveling with her was delightful and she came through as a true spirit sister. She taught me how to focus, and inspired business strategies and creative ideas with her stimulating questions to the Young Living leaders. Being around her was quite a lesson since my mind does not work anything like hers. I was truly thankful.

Caleb's story was a gem. He attributed his metamorphosis to meeting Wifey at his first weeklong essential oil training with Gary Young in Dallas in 1997. Wifey helped facilitate the seminar of 800 people. Three people were assigned to a massage table working on one another while Gary demonstrated the techniques on stage. I know about this because I was there as well. Anyway, Wifey had four people on Caleb's massage table, his two brothers and mother, and she helped them layer the oils on the body that lay on the table. Caleb remembered Wifey quite well because he was from a very strict religious family background and Wifey, simply put, was not. Wifey has a beautiful tattoo on her back of a naked woman holding symbols of light along with other powerful sacred symbols with deep meaning. Caleb was totally taken aback by her tattoo and the gears in his mind were churning as to how he would interact with her. The oils can change things around quite fast and his brother was having a major emotional release while Wifey stuck by to facilitate the healing and release. A seed was planted inside of Caleb during this experience and he kept shedding his old belief system and blooming from within from that day on. He enjoyed talking and joking about how absurd his old belief system used to be.

Caleb was a great complement to our little posse. He was a computer expert with lots of clever ideas for strategizing the most efficient ways to promote your own business. I happened to be one of the lucky recipients of his valuable wisdom.

After being hypnotized in our time warp loop by one another's company, one of us decided to snap out of it and check the time. It was time to meet our cabdriver and venture back to the ship. I enjoyed a lovely evening show watching dancing and singing to show tunes. Then I met Mary Hardy and the gang at the pool on deck 11 and we performed our nightly vortex ritual.

Wifey, Londin, Brent, and I decided to start earlier the next day in Antigua, head for a reef, and snorkel. Our cabdriver, Joseph the Coat of Many Colors, dropped us off at another beautiful crystal blue ocean with a Clorox white beach, where the snorkel excursion people where patiently waiting for us. We were late and waited for a small boat to take us out to a reef. While Wifey and I waited, a beautiful young black Virgin Island woman began admiring Wifey's body.

"I love your body—are you black?" she asked.

We laughed and laughed at her astute observation. Wifey has more of an African body than a white one. She has always thought that she was a black girl trapped in a white girl's skin. She has a small upper body and a sexy bubble butt that the natives marvel at. The Virgin Island African descendants fell in love with Wifey. It was entertainingly humorous to witness the native men and women admire her.

Soon we were aboard a small speedboat with our new captain *Fantastic Plastic* at the helm, while he aggressively flirted with Wifey and she did not mind in the least. As the island tourist facilitators would have it we had to trade Fantastic Plastic in for the main captain, *Godjewel*. We called him *God* for short. God brought us to a beautiful reef that we had all to ourselves. This was a wonderful experience for me to reintroduce myself to snorkeling without being afraid after my last encounter with a breast lump. I swam on top of the water and did not dive down so I would not put pressure on my face, and still had a very entertaining view of the colorful fish feeding and swimming around the coral reef. God kept a close eye and took great care of us, as you would expect. Upon our return, Fantastic Plastic became reacquainted with Wifey while we waited for Joseph the Coat of Many Colors to bring our posse back to the ship.

Joseph the Coat of Many Colors sent Berry in his place. We asked,

"Berry of...?" and he replied,

"Just Berry."

Berry brought us safely back to the ship so we could start all over again the next day.

We got another late start with a long, engaging breakfast on the ship in St. Lucia. This day consisted of Wifey, Londin, and I praying for a magickal, spontaneous day. Brent stayed behind and was busy catching up with his long-distance healing sessions with his clients. We did not see Caleb because he went with the large Young Living group on another excursion.

Wifey, Londin, and I asked for an easy, non-tourist, magickal day with the rain forest included. We ventured off the ship and into the lion's den, where the local excursion sharks were feeding. We refused a boat trip with 28 drunken snorkeling tourists and spent some time talking to a tall, dark gentleman about a cab ride around the island. We explained to him what we were looking for and it was definitely not the typical request he had encountered before. We asked to have a day away from tourists, a spiritual experience in the rain forest, and a personal experience with the locals. Our patient tourist info guy's name was *Easy*; it was not his day to drive but his turn to promote his company and the other drivers for the day. After listening carefully to our request he decided he would grant us our wishes and be our guide for the day. This was a highly unusual request and not really lucrative for the company, but he felt like meeting our challenge anyway.

Easy had the magickal name we prayed for as well as a delightful temperament to be our most gracious host. He drove us away from the main tourist areas as requested. Our first stop was on the side of the road, where a woman was cutting up young coconuts. They were delicious—the young meat tasted and felt like pudding as well as being a very healthy food, rich in nutrients. The coconut van was parked in front of a sign that read *Emergency Banana Recovery Unit*. I did not ask Easy to clarify this sign, I just used my imagination; does this unit save bananas or are you recovered after slipping on a banana peel?

IT'S NOT WEIRD ANYMORE

On our way to the rain forest we witnessed a very bad accident. Locals risk passing on blind curves and are completely surprised when a car is head-on in the lane they are passing in. I said a silent prayer for the people involved and felt grateful it was not me this time.

Easy brought us to a rain forest trail and Londin, Wifey, and I hiked the trail, found a clearing, performed the vortex ritual, and encountered no one. We enjoyed the trees, plants, and wind while Easy waited at the trailhead with his car.

On the road again, we wound our way to a private waterfall on an organic farm. Easy continuously asked if this was what we wanted for an experience. We told him it exceeded our expectations and we were very happy with his choices. He seemed to love hearing how much we were enjoying ourselves. We had a lovely time perched underneath the waterfall in our bathing suits while bantering with our young guide who came with the excursion while Easy patiently waited for our return.

Now the best part of the whole adventure was ahead. Easy brought us to his home to meet his wife and children. We were so touched and felt privileged and the feeling was mutual coming from Easy because he was having a very pleasant, unusual day himself. His wife, Margaret, made us fresh-squeezed grapefruit juice that tasted yummy and sweet. We talked with Margaret while she held the new addition to their family, one-and-a-half-year-old Hanna, on her lap. The back porch overlooking the small bay and beautiful view across the island was where our visit took place. Easy's son joined us after returning home from school. Time passed while we experienced a full day of adventure and headed back to the ship. Everyone including Easy felt completely satisfied. The conversation on the ride back was Easy probing us about ways to create a business, taking tourists away from the tourist areas.

As I walked back to the ship I saw Easy kicked back with a very pleasant smile on his face sitting with his bosses. He got up and approached me and waved his boss over to talk to me about our day. I thanked his boss and said Easy was a magnificent host for creating our day. I believe Easy felt complete after that.

Wifey, Londin, and I caught up with Caleb on board and listened to him describe his long bus ride with a couple hundred Young Living oilers. Everyone seemed to complain about the four-hour roundtrip bus ride with barely a land excursion and many tourist shops. We knew then that we had made the best choice in having our spontaneous day with Easy.

Brent appeared satisfied with his day as well, catching up with his clients. I asked him to work some of his magick on me and he graciously accepted. That evening he spent time asking my body, mind, and spirit permission on several levels for the work to take place. He said I would be releasing for a few days and to just allow it to happen.

Our last land day in Barbados began with a very long, engaging breakfast again. Our posse consisted of Londin, Brent, Wifey, and I deciding how we wanted our day to go. We heard about swimming with giant sea turtles and thought that sounded good. We were directed to a place called the Blue Monkey. It turned out to be an open-air beach restaurant with many touristy things to do on the beach. Brent's main focus was finding out if he could rent a small Hobie Cat sailboat. Londin, Wifey, and I hung out on the beach with familiar faces from our Young Living cruise while we waited for Brent to finish up his investigation. Caleb had been on the beach for hours before we arrived and gave us tourist tips. It was easy to rent snorkel gear and swim out to the turtles without a boat. The best way to see them was when the tourist boat threw breadcrumbs for feeding since there was not a reef to swim around for seafood.

Brent came back smiling and had scored a small Hobie Cat that could take three. I easily chose to stay behind since I sailed for many years and know the thrill. In addition I was not that keen on speed because it was the last day on land, same as the last cruise that ended with the crash. I felt comfortable socializing on the beach with Caleb. I did not feel motivated to swim out to the turtles without a reef to admire and no guarantee that the boat would throw crumbs and I may or may not catch a glimpse of the magnificent creatures. Caleb expressed hunger, so I accompanied him to the Blue Monkey and we ordered food together. We invited a mother and daughter essential oil business team to join us and once again there were more moments lost in time with interesting conversation. I watched a speeding sailboat with rainbow-colored sails race by in the distance and thought, *I bet I know who is on that vessel.*

It took some time to get served since the Blue Monkey was extremely busy. Brent, Londin, and Wifey joined us at our table after their excursion and yes; the little craft with the rainbow-colored sails was theirs.

Brent seemed to be studying me from across the table and asked me to move over to an empty table with him. He began moving my energy and taking something away. I stood for a brief moment and started to get lightheaded and dizzy and requested to sit down. The diners were watching me and wondering what in the world was taking place. Everything went black as I leaned against the wall and blacked out. I was not gone for long and heard Brent's gentle, encouraging voice bring me back while he continued to use his hands to move a particular energy out of me. He said he was guided to take me back to the day of the accident and pull the grief from my body. How interesting—this happened to be the exact time of day and the last day of the cruise as before. Nothing is weird anymore.

I came away knowing that I could begin to recover my inner strength again. I believe we are all surrounded with many angels in physical form as well as nonphysical. I have truly come full circle with my year-and-one-quarter-long adventure.

I was ready to return home to my beloved Peter, whom I have missed deeply. It feels good to miss him; although we both felt this time apart would be beneficial for us.

IT'S NOT WEIRD ANYMORE

~ 41 ~

I looked forward to connecting with Delilah to hear about Egypt and feel the new energy in Seattle after the Dalai Lama's visit. Delilah had a wonderfully magickal experience with her group of 27. To be brief, she and her group of dancers performed on the top deck of their Nile cruise for four nights. Her entourage was given a private showing in the Kings Chamber of the great Cheops pyramid, where her group was invisibly guided to perform different spontaneous rituals. Delilah said what took place was pretty wild and of course not weird anymore.

Upon Delilah's arrival at SeaTac airport, she was taking the escalator down and passed the Dalai Lama going up. When he was in close range he started a spontaneous kind of Shiva dance posture, looking animated as he gazed deep into her eyes with recognition while he glided by. Yes, I believe the energies have shifted once again, moving closer to the light and my circle of friends and I played our part.

Note: The resource section has updates that go beyond the end of the narrative, with my commentary in italics, as well as more entertaining wisdom and observation. Don't miss the Origin of the Belly Dance, a most beautiful, poetic tale about the story of creation in the belly dance section. Enjoy.

Resources

Resources: All resource web links can be found at:
www.ItsNotWeirdAnymore.com with the username: *itsnotweirdanymore* and the password: *iamlove* to gain access.

 Laura's note: Several of the resource practitioners are local to the Seattle area and their specific healing technique can be found all over the globe. You can easily find the technique in your area with a quick Internet search. Some practitioners will even travel to teach and work their craft.

LAURA LEGERE

Acupuncture

Acupuncture is a healing art and science that teaches how to see the entire human being in body-mind-spirit wholeness, how to recognize the process of health and illness, and how to restore lost health to an individual. This system originated 5,000 years ago in India and was used to prevent illness by helping to create and maintain good health. The Chinese developed the art of acupuncture medicine as we know it today—a complex system of examination, diagnosis, and treatment. It is also used for pain relief and pre and post surgery recovery.

Kitty Wittkower graduated from NIAOM Acupuncture School in 1999, where she completed her MA degree and did clinical training. She added acupuncture to her yoga teaching practice to better serve the needs of her clients, helping people overcome injuries and other health challenges, bringing their bodies and minds back into balance.

Kitty's treatments may include suggestions of yoga and meditation practices, when appropriate, to help clients become more aware of how to heal themselves. When dietary issues are addressed she prefers Ayurvedic dietary recommendations because of the variety and flexibility.

Kitty's yoga training focuses on asana technique, with a special emphasis on therapeutics, for injury and illness.

Kitty has practiced yoga since the early 1980s and in 1992 was certified in the Iyengar method. Recently completing another teacher training, with Siva Rae in Seattle in 2005, she continues her education with other yoga luminaries that include: Dona Holleman, Dharma Mitra, Ana Forest, Sharon Gannon, David Life, Gary Kraftstow, Kathleen Hunt, and most recently Les Leventhal.

Laura's note: I have watched many people attempt yoga for the first time and get discouraged by joining a big class with a teacher who does not assist them with what their body can comfortably do. They then conclude that yoga is not for them. There are many different kinds of yoga and teachers and I encourage you to investigate further. Yoga keeps you young, healthy, and flexible and Kitty is a great teacher who can assist you on whatever level your body will allow.

Adam Kadmon Body (24 Key DNA strands)

From the beginning of time, prophecies and legends have spoken of humankind evolving into a *God-like* being. Our modern culture and media are full of tales and myths of superheroes or humans that possess certain powers and abilities beyond most. They are stories that we have grown up with as children, stories that have always permeated our culture and society, yet only ever relegated to the realms of fairy tales and fantasy.

For thousands of years the *Universal Kabbalah* has referred to this phenomenon as the prophecy of the *Adam Kadmon*, which literally translates into *God Human*. Throughout their tradition the Mystery Schools have often spoken of the *Great Work*, which is defined as the unification of the body, mind, and soul with the Spirit. This unification is the ultimate transformation of the self into one's highest potential being, an exalted state of divine awareness and consciousness.

In the tradition of the Universal Kabbalah, Adam Kadmon is the name used for this God-like being. It refers to the legend of Adam as the first man and woman (Adam meaning *many* in reference to the entire human race) and our return to that state of being. The Kabbalah also refers to the Kadmon, meaning *completion*. Therefore, Adam Kadmon is a return to our beginning, but a return with all the knowledge and wisdom of the physical world integrated into our physical and spiritual beings.

Laura's note: I mentioned early on in the narrative that I received the Adam Kadmon activation and believe it played a part in my accelerated healing process. I received the 22-strand DNA activation first and later had two more strands activated to make up the Adam Kadmon body. According to the Mystery School ten years ago most people had one or two strands activated and use five to ten percent of their brain capacity. How much of your brain you are using is directly related to how much of your DNA is activated. The activation activates the master cell of the pineal gland, which holds the blueprint of who you are and what you came here to do. According to the Mystery School, when our DNA is fully activated it looks like the Tree of Life, spins clockwise and has a blue core in the center. I believe this pattern is in everything and we are the Tree of Life. The Tree of Life is a map directing us to God/Goddess all that is and we have the blueprint within ourselves to guide us on the pathway home.

The Adam Kadmon Activation is offered through the Mystery School. See Mystery School in this resource directory as well as a further explanation of the Kabbalah under Kabbalah.

Art

The Fremont Arts Council in Seattle believes that art is essential to community. And even more: that great art creates community itself—through stewardship, a sense of belonging, and collective participation.

Our vision is of a Fremont that's a fun, interesting, and beautiful place to live, to work, and to visit. And, of course, one that's for everyone—whether big and small, professional artist or beginner—to make great art in.

What We Do:
We use creativity to build a stronger community. We believe in art as an integral part of everyday life. We promote diversity of viewpoints, backgrounds & art forms.

Our Principles:
   We accept fiscal responsibility for our decisions.
   We believe participation & equal access to power is essential.
   We honor integrity.
   We respect our work/play space & environment. Recycling is part of our art.
   We support growth that balances our resources, tradition & intent.
   We communicate effectively both internally & externally. We believe in each other's goodwill and working together.
   We welcome everyone, regardless of who they are and what they think or believe.
   We uphold an ethic of equality: we support and celebrate human dignity and diversity.
   Our Goal is to use consensus decision-making and information sharing, so as many people as possible can be involved in the creative process.

Belly Dancing

Visionary Dance Productions
   Delilah is an internationally acclaimed belly dance performer and instructor. She grew up in Southern California, learning the dance form as it was passed on and popularized in this country by first- and second-generation immigrants from Lebanon, Armenia, Iraq, Syria, Iran, Egypt, Israel, Turkey, Morocco, and Greece. Her years of devoted study and practice have led her to become one of the foremost teachers and innovators in the field of belly dance today. She is widely known for her breathtaking and deeply inspiring performances.
   When Delilah was 18, belly dance was fast becoming an American phenomenon. As thousands of women absorbed this dance by way of diverse cultural experience, a new style of American Belly Dance evolved. Delilah is an active part of this transformation. While dancing in ethnic nightclubs, fairs, theater productions, and folk-style house parties for almost 20 years, she has learned many different styles of dance, and has also learned about music, food, customs, religions, politics, and people. Her belly dance experience fuels her interest in studying the fields of mythology, archeology, history, women's studies, bio-ecology, psychology, healing practices, and other movement forms such as tai

chi, yoga, modern dance, and movement therapy.

Delilah currently has her own video/dance studio called V.D.P. (Visionary Dance Productions) Studios, located in Seattle, Washington. There she teaches and hosts other instructors from all over the world in a fusion of Middle Eastern arts, music, and dance. She has a unique collection of instruction DVDs, music, and belly dance attire. She has held yearly Visionary Belly Dance Retreats in Hawaii since 1992; this annual retreat is now frequented by dancers from all over the world.

Dahlia Moon has been teaching and performing various styles of belly dance for over a decade. Before moving to the Seattle area in 2003, she taught and performed regularly in Arabic and Turkish restaurants in Osaka, Japan for two years. Prior to living in Asia, Dahlia performed solo and troupe work throughout the Pacific Northwest.

Dahlia is fortunate to have been born into a family of musicians. She has been surrounded by live music and song her entire life. Being a musician herself allows her to transform music into movement with expertise and ease. Dahlia has a BS in anthropology and has also studied other forms of dance, such as ballet, jazz, modern, flamenco, Japanese, salsa, and ballroom throughout her life, but has a special place in her heart for Raqs Sharqi and Dance Orientale (Egyptian Belly Dance). Blessed with a talent for music and dance, Dahlia performs with unaffected intensity, skillful grace, and sheer joy.

Elisa Gamal took her first belly dance class in 1987, and made her professional debut to the stages of Seattle in 1994. Highlights of her career include winning numerous solo and group awards, including the 1999 Belly Dance USA and 2006 Seven Veils Champion titles, being featured on the cover of *Jareeda* magazine, and performing as a guest with the Belly Dance Superstars on their first US tour.

Elisa is a board member and vice president of Middle East Arts International. She enjoys an active performance schedule, appearing at several Seattle area venues, dance festivals, and cultural events, including the Northwest Folklife Festival and Arab Festival.

A sought-after instructor and intuitive, supportive, and effective coach, Elisa has watched several of her current and past students gain national recognition and win trophies and titles in nearly every major US belly dance competition. "Belly Dance is my passion and my inspiration, my solace and my release, my source of renewal and profound joy."

Laura Rose is known for drama and intensity in her dance. Her years of studying theater and character development have contributed to her range and artistry through belly dance. She has toured extensively with belly dance revues and also has had plenty of dance troupe experience where she has to be a quick study at on-the-spot pantomime and choreography. All this has attributed to her wealth of understanding about how it's done.

The Origin of the Belly Dance

This story was channeled to me through my friend Maggie Price, may she rest in peace. It is from Selene, the Moon Goddess. I have a memory of temple dancing and felt as if I was back at it again while I danced with Delilah and seemed to recognize all the women I danced with on a regular basis. I asked Maggie what was the origin of the belly dance and this is what transpired. This story was transcribed from a cassette tape as it was given to me in one long sentence.

There are so many of us that would like to speak to you. There are energies from the stars, of the moon, beginnings of your dance, of yourselves, of how it all came about. That you are who you are and you do what you do. You have been interested in a form of dance that is part of creation, that which brought the earth into being. I have been chosen to speak with you, my name is Selene, I am a bright and shining star person as each of you are.

In the beginning as the tone was given and creation began, it began through motion, motion of energies, sparkling energies, crashing throughout the universe, crashing throughout the all. As from the great void we came, into the great void we went, gathering momentum, shining, dimming and shining again. As earth took on its form in the formlessness of the all there was a below and there was an above and in the spinning and rotation of those energies there came into being the bluing of all things within and upon the earth. The tone, as the energies spun, began to produce color, the colors of the rainbow, and in the beginning and you've asked for the beginning as the rainbow was seen at times it undulated and this in regard to the earth is your form of dance about which you inquire. It became most noticeable as the tone turning to color danced as to what is called the aurora borealis, the northern lights; which was formed first before all else, before any planet, before any continent, before any earth form. While there were only the waters of the deep, still there was tone and there was color. As the poles began to spin as the dervish, they spun materials outward much as a spindle of yarn would gather energies and form an orb that was called earth. The tone that became color remained at the north and is still seen as the aurora borealis. But the earth was her own first dancer, wore her own beautiful colored rainbow, danced her own dance and as you who were particles of energy joined together on this new planet and watched her and proceeded to assist her, to form her land-masses and later her civilizations, her flora and fauna, her animals, her beings the two-leggeds. As all of this transpired each in your own way had your own form, your own tone, your own color, as this was observed by various tribes of humans or communities of humans, individuals who were placed here and there who found each other and gathered together. There were rituals that were performed and always a dance, always a dance, always a dance. The dancers became aware when they could see color, which was not in the beginning, no one could see color, everything was in grays, blacks and whites and everything was shaded, so that there was nothing that was visible to the human eye or to the eye of the beings that inhabited the planet in the beginning.

They say that animals cannot see color, animals can see color, it is only because people think that animals are lesser than they are, that they cannot see color. Animals have seen color long before humans saw color. The nature kingdom came into color and the animals and the birds and the fishes of the sea could see and understand the tones, which brought this color about. They helped to produce the color because they knew the tones, the birds knew the singing tones, and the whales and the dolphins knew the depth tones and the water tones. The grasses and the leaves knew the rustling tones and they produced these tones and they took on these colors. Eventually when man heard himself for the first time and uttered a guttural tone from his own vocal cords that had been mute, which he did not know how to use, he discovered that as that tone arose from his throat that his physical eyes began to behold certain colors in certain areas and he was amazed, he was struck dumb, he could speak again, he could not speak, but then he hadn't been speaking, it was so shocking to him, and he so enjoyed the feeling of the tone that he uttered it again. He uttered it over and over and over again until his eyes were fully opened and the veil peeled away and he could see the full color spectrum of what lay before him and he was amazed again. He became aware of other beings close in proximity to him and in his joy and jubilation he ran to share this wonderful news, and in that sharing he encouraged others to experiment with their own tones. The magic as he called it that came from inside, the magic that came from inside, the magic that comes from inside through the heart that opens the orbs, which are eyes.

Until presently, after the beyond of course all people were seeing colors and then nature began to teach them how to use these colors. Those who lived furthest north beheld the northern lights and the skies were clear then and the northern lights could be seen throughout the entire northern hemisphere of this great planet. Civilization began to spring forth and we are not conveying this historically or properly, but I am a storyteller tonight, Selene is telling a story.

On the great land-mass of Lemuria there were those with faraway memories, memories of other stars of other planets and they knew colors and tones that were not present on this planet. It is only now that you are being prepared to peel away further layers from your eyes so that you may see more color through learning more tones. There are more tones than you have ever heard as a human in this body today. Therefore there is color for every tone. You dance the dance and you dance color and you dance tone and you bring them together and you are the northern lights, you are the aurora borealis, you are the reflection of the fish swimming in deep water, you are the opalescence of that fish, you are the opalescence of the pearl, you are the opalescence of the inside of the shell that is so beautiful. You are all these things and the dance that you dance came from the center of the earth; it came from the great void of creation into the great void that became earth. On this great continent, on this original land-mass called Lemuria there were some very high beings, as I said before with memories of other planets, of other stars, of other colors and tones. These were very high sacred beings who began the spiritual teachings on Lemuria that later became Atlantis. It was while they were on Lemuria, before that land-mass broke apart, that they in bare body form took on the luminescence or colors, the beautiful pale pastel colors of their each and several planets and stars from which they came. This was their ceremony, their ritual, it was their dance. You now call it the belly dance and that is because in the beginning there dropped into the great void and into the center of the great void the tone that represents the naval of the earth and that naval runs from pole to pole.

Countries claim to be the beginning of civilization, countries claim that they know where the center of civilization is and indeed they do for their era, for their era. They do not understand that millions and millions of years prior was the navel of the earth implanted and it became the axis of the earth upon which the earth turns as she does her own dance. This is why as you do what you call your belly dance you expose yourselves as much as your society permits and in the center of your belly lies your naval, your axis, the axis of the dance around which you spin, around which you move, which is the center of creation and is your center where your umbilical cord to your great mother began and ended.

As the dance began in this area of Lemuria that broke away and became the great civilization of Atlantis the dance had already been established. It was danced with no veils, with no covering save the varied colors that emanated from the bodies of the dancers representing the colors and tones of those stars, of those planets, of those systems from whence they came; from this galaxy and galaxies further away. It was done in great reverence and great holiness and always, always the naval was recognized as the center of the dance. All consecration of any of these beings to their source of power, the one creator, the one could only be given through, the expression of the naval as the center of the great body of the earth, the center of the great body of the human, the center of the great body of the one, and all tone and all reverence was given to the naval.

Later in Atlantis as the dance developed there were jewels that were placed in the naval. Jewels that reflected the color of the sun's rays, of the moons reflection of the sun's rays, so that even done at night the fluorescence of the dancer's body which still held the reflection of the essence of the colors of the stars and the planets from which they came could be seen, and all the energies through which they had passed covered their bodies. The center, the jewel in the naval, gathered all of these colors together and as they danced they created and sent messages of joy, peace, love and harmony throughout the all of creation. These dances were done by the edge of a great water so that there was more reflection and more reflection and more reflection and it rippled outward and could be seen from other stars in the galaxy and from other planets in the galaxy. Thus communication was never broken with the stars and the planets. Indeed as you dance now, the most sacred dance of all dances, remember always that the message goes out from the naval and depending on the colors you are drawn to wear you are connecting the stars and the planets from which you in your various lifetimes have visited and have come from and because you have a naval you can be seen as human and are known as beings from the earth and of the earth. Never turn your back on this dance; it has been danced in the most sacred of temples in every civilization; there is no civilization that can lay claim to this dance; it is more than international, it is intergalactic and you must never ever forget this. It has been commercialized, it has been desecrated, it has gone through all manner of trauma of being put down and of being lifted up again. At this point in time those who misuse it suffer the consequences, those who misunderstand it are held where they are until they begin to understand what it is about. It is the most powerful tool that those of you who have passed it on from civilization to civilization of which you are one and who now still carry the memory of it from past lifetimes. It is the most powerful tool which you have to communicate with those whom you now call extraterrestrials, where they see you, they recognize you and they know who you are, and because they recognize who you are, you will draw to you those of your own from other stars, from other planets.

Be always aware that the earth is still turning on her axis, that the aurora borealis is still weaving her magic spell, doing her own dance and the dances she creates are amazing, amazing not only in their color but in their formations. Every time you do a dance you are carrying this planet earth further and further into the 5th, 6th and 7th dimensions, for the design of the dance as it is created spontaneously without planning, sets up in the turning in color, sets up a tone that is harmonious and in tune with other tones that are emitted by the earth to carry the earth and all of humanity into higher and higher overtones. You are doing a service through all of humanity as you dance knowingly, being fully aware of the importance of the dance.

Every culture has its own dance; every culture is just as important as any other culture. Those of you with the memory of creation do the dance of creation, are still doing the dance of creation and will never stop, never stop. Blessed are you who are on the path, blessed are your hands as they simulate the dance as you work the energies of those who need you for the movements are the same. As your hands move, you're moving the energies in the same ways as you move your body in the dance, so that you are creating within the individual who receives your blessing through your hands the opening of the channels which have been blocked to the dance and to their own awareness of creation. You dance with your hands on the bodies of those who come to you to be assisted, to be healed, to be helped, to be opened and the patterns are the same and you continue to create. I have come to you tonight in particular to remove any doubt that you might have about anything. Nothing can stand in the way of the motion of the dance. Doubt comes from the ego, it is nothing, it is not even existed, you cannot claim it, it has no essence. Love does have essence and that is all that needs to be claimed. You cannot claim fear, it has no essence, it is of the ego. You cannot say you are afraid, soon you will not even to able to form those words with your mouth because your mouth will not form the words, because those thoughts have no body, have no essence, have no identity, no being, no fullness, nothing, they are of nothing as is the ego.

You are changing, you are turning, you are whirling, you are dancing, you are the dance and you are the dancer, you are creation itself. Let this never go unheard, never. Dance to the moon, dance to the stars, dance to the sun, dance for the people, dance in the streets, dance in the water, dance on the grass, dance for the animals, dance for the trees, dance for joy and dance for sorrow. Cause a transformation to complete itself again and again and be transformed by the very act of transformation. Watch the magic before your eyes, dance for those you love, dance for those you do not love, dance, create, spin around your naval. Appreciate who you are and who you have always been.

Thank you for this opportunity and on behalf of the others who understand the creativity and understand the dance.

August 1995 channeling by Maggie Price

I thanked and blessed Selene for bringing me this phenomenal story of the origin of the belly dance. At the very end of the channeled tape there was a faint heartbeat that became louder and louder until it seemed to blast the room. I believe this heartbeat to be the Great Mother Earth herself. I have read this story aloud many times and have never been able to read it with dry eyes. It has always moved me to tears.

Maggie was my spiritual mentor for 16 years and channeled whomever I would benefit to speak with in the moment. She claimed to be the reincarnation of Madam Blavaski, a famous Russian psychic medium who founded the

LAURA LEGERE

Theosophical Society formed in the 1870s. Looking at photos of Blavaski and Maggie they almost look identical.

Belly Dance Middle Eastern Music

House of Tarab *(Laura's Tribute Dinner Band)*
"Finally a Middle Eastern recording by artist with something to say! House of Tarab's first recording employs original arrangements of classical pieces making them fresh and fun. The addition of several pieces of the chorus really adds a great dynamic. Talented musicians playing acoustic instruments with taste and soul. Great for dancing and listening."
Mark Bell of Helm, CA, Musician and Grammy Winner

House of Tarab's newly released CD is played with a better than authentic zest for life. Salah Ali from Baghdad plays a sensuous solo on his violin that all dancers swoon over. David McGrath's ney playing is superb and soulful, Stephen Elaimy is a second-generation oud player from Palestine who has toured with Delilah in Korea. American Jane Hall rocks on Riq, and Erik Brown from DC plays solid on tabla. These musicians have exceptional chemistry together.

Laura's note: I give admiration and thanks to the beautiful dancers, dances and music performed at my Tribute Dinner.

Bio-Identical Hormones & Naturopathy

The Wiley Protocol formulation and manner of dosing bio-mimetic HRT started out as a *thought experiment* in a book called *Sex, Lies and Menopause* by medical writer and researcher T.S. Wiley. In the book, Wiley asked the question "If hormone replacement was made of real bio-mimetic hormones and dosed to mimic the ups and downs of the hormone blood levels in a normal menstrual cycle in a 20-year-old woman, would all of the symptoms and disease states of aging decline or even, disappear?" Well, to her surprise and many others, the logic holds—because it was the rhythm that was always missing in other regimens. The Wiley Protocol is a trademarked, patent-pending delivery system consisting of biomimetic estradiol and progesterone dosed to mimic the natural hormones produced by your body when you were 20 years old.

Dr. Lucinda Messer ND graduated in 1994 from Bastyr University with a doctorate in naturopathic medicine, and has specialty training in several areas: women's health issues, allergies, NAET, natural hormone replacement, and anti-aging medicine.

Dr. Messer is a member of the American Association of Naturopathic Physicians, the Washington Association of Naturopathic Physicians, the Anti-Aging Medical Society (AAM), and the American Society of Aesthetic Mesotherapy.

She is a member of the Bastyr University Speaker's Bureau and speaks on several health issues, representing Bastyr. She has contributed to several publications on hormonal issues, especially on the thyroid.

Dr. Messer's Goddess Sanctuary

A day to yourself or with a group of friends to relax, enjoy, and experience the divinity of the Goddess Sanctuary... Includes: yoga, sweat lodge, infrared sauna or spa, massage, or facial and a body wrap of your choice! Plus foot-detox bath, reflexology, and more!

Retreats: All-day or half-day retreats available!

Treatments: FREE! Ozonated Jacuzzi or IR sauna session with purchase of any therapy!

Massage Therapy

Facials Therapy

Specialty Body Wraps: All wraps include exfoliation (brush or salt), Wrap, and body moisturizer.

Signature "Sabai" hot stone therapy, detoxifying lymphatic drainage, deep tissue, relaxation/Swedish therapy, cranial sacral, and reflexology

Chiropractic

Koren Specific Technique, or KST for short, is a relatively new style of chiropractic, although some of the components have been around for more than 70 years. In 2003 Tedd Koren, an American chiropractor, put the final touches to the technique he had been developing and started teaching it in 2005.

All chiropractors, of whatever persuasion, do three things.

1. They detect subluxations, the misalignments that compromise the nervous system.
2. They decide how the subluxations need to be corrected.
3. They adjust the subluxations.

KST is no different. It does all three things, it's just that the way it is done is very different from the styles of chiropractic we already practice and are accustomed to. The methods KST uses are more toward the esoteric or vitalistic end of the spectrum as opposed to the exoteric or mechanistic end. In fact it uses some very cutting-edge neurological and physiological discoveries. KST is a very gentle, yet powerful, result-oriented technique.

Dr. Steve Polenz

"I had never experienced anything as wonderful as my first chiropractic adjustment. Chiropractic allowed me to recover from all of my pain and injuries, and improved my digestion and overall health. I get adjusted regularly to keep myself as healthy as possible." Dr. Steve Polenz

Dr. Steve's focus in practice is based on his own experiences as a patient of chiropractic. The day he discovered how to properly combine Koren chiropractic with nutritional healing and emotional work was the day he was able to go from helping his patients feel better to helping them truly become healthy and alive again.

Codex Alimentarius

Codex Alimentarius, established in 1962 as a UN trade commission, serves corporate greed with no interest in health or consumer protection. The World Health Organization says Codex Alimentarius "has not made a contribution in human health in its 42 years of existence."

Codex Alimentarius sponsors are Big Pharma (drug companies that make huge profits on unnecessarily expensive drugs), Big Medica (pro-illness industry thrives when you and/or family are ill), Big Chema (profitable toxic chemicals used on food and fields, including deadly pesticides banned in the US), Big Agribiz (industrial farms use antibiotics, drugs, hormones to increase profits) and Big Biotechna (creates dangerous untested Genetically Modified Organisms or GMOs) planned to become legal worldwide unlabeled). Codex Alimentarius has no actual legal standing BUT exerts a lot of influence since it is used by the World Trade Organization (WTO) to decide trade disputes. Codex-compliant countries win automatically regardless of the merits of the case. Devastating trade sanctions result, so the US is now racing to destroy protective laws to clear the way to "HARMonize" with Codex.

This is what Codex has in store for us:

1. Declare nutrients toxins so Codex will supposedly protect us from them.
2. Ban virtually all-natural health options.
3. All effective, high-potency nutrients will be illegal with or without a prescription.
4. Only a few ultra low-dose nutrients will be legal, all others banned while deadly drugs are sold unopposed.
5. Dangerous growth stimulants (hormones) mandatory in all meat and milk (e.g., Monsanto's BGH).
6. Deadly banned pesticides permitted in your food.
7. Untested, unlabeled Franken-food in your kitchen. (GMOs – Genetically

Modified Organisms)
8. Free-radical rich irradiated food.
9. Widespread under-nutrition resulting in increased cancer, diabetes, heart disease, stroke, autoimmune diseases, depression, obesity, autism – the list is endless.
10. Weak and meaningless *Organic Farming* standards allowing dangerous drugs and chemicals in so-called *Organic* food.

Codex Alimentarius is global in scope and affects all World Trade Organization member countries (including the USA) despite disinformation to the contrary. Codex is already being implemented, standard by standard, and needs our action to protect our food and health choices now. Healthy people are bad for the most powerful industries in the world: Big Pharma and Big Medica. Adulteration of food and elimination of nutrients means people cannot get healthy or stay that way as huge profits result for the adulterators in the process.

We the people of the USA thereby revoke any influence Codex Alimentarius has in the past, present, and future of our health freedoms and defeat all bills before Congress clearing the way for "HARMonization" with Codex.

What can you do? See Health Freedom *in this resource directory.*

Colon Hydrotherapy

Colon Hydrotherapy is the cleansing of the large intestine (colon) through the administration of water, herbal solutions, enzymes, and other natural substances. Colon hydrotherapy is a method of detoxifying the body through the removal of accumulated waste from the colon. Detoxification increases the efficiency of the body's natural healing abilities and can be helpful when combating an illness or as a general preventive health measure and part of a routine internal hygiene regimen.

Gayle Palms is a certified instructor of colon therapy and member of I-ACT (International Association of Colon Therapists). She is passionate about improving the overall health of her clients through colon therapy and education. Gayle has been administering colon hydrotherapy (colonics) since 1997 as well as training, instructing, and certifying new practitioners. She is also an herbalist and EPFX Quantum Bio-Feedback Practitioner.

Gayle is very skilled, calm, patient, and has an instinctive ability to help you relax. It takes a special person to perform a colonic and Gayle has the right qualities for this practice.

LAURA LEGERE

Contact Talk Radio

Cameron Steele Co-Host of *Live with Cameron and Davindia* 9 to 11 a.m. PST Monday thru Friday on 1150 AM.

In 1996 Cameron began forming the vision for CONTACT Talk Radio. With a background in TV and radio, he saw the need for a medium that would bring information and resources to people that would improve their lives, assist in their personal and spiritual journeys, and contribute to creating wholeness for the world. An energetic and vibrant free spirit, Cam has hosted television shows such as *After Hours* in Vancouver, BC and *New Age Northwest* in Seattle. With an eclectic background of blue and white-collar experiences, he brings a sense of the common everyman to listeners as he invites them in his warm, disarming, and no-nonsense way to be extraordinary.

Davindia Anjanet Steele

Davindia's background has been largely spent in the real estate industry. She realized early on that her motivation in the industry was solely community building and assisting people in finding a place where they belong. Though reluctant in joining husband Cameron on air March of 2002 to co-host the show, it did not take long for Davindia to embrace the opportunity to build community on a mass scale through this unique forum. With an adept ability to ask the questions that get to the heart of the matter, she is able to identify the gems of insight the show's guests bring, and she connects the listeners to that message. Davindia has an enormous heart, and her compassion flows across the airwaves. She has a passion for social justice and environmental awareness that she brings to the show.

Cranial Sacral Therapy

by Michael Kern, DO., R.C.S.T., M.I.Cr.A., N.D.

Life expresses itself as motion. At a deep level of our physiological functioning all healthy, living tissues subtly *breathe* with the motion of life—a phenomenon that produces rhythmic impulses that can be palpated by sensitive hands. The presence of these subtle rhythms in the body was discovered by osteopath Dr. William Sutherland over 100 years ago, after he had a remarkable insight while examining the specialized articulations of cranial bones. Contrary to popular belief Dr. Sutherland realized that cranial sutures were, in fact, designed to express small degrees of motion. He undertook many years of research, during which he demonstrated the existence of this motion and eventually concluded it is essentially produced by the body's inherent life force, which he referred to as the *Breath of Life*. Furthermore, Dr. Sutherland discovered that the motion of cranial bones he first discovered is closely connected to subtle movements that involve a network of interrelated tissues and fluids at the core of the body;

including cerebrospinal fluid (the "sap in the tree"), the central nervous system, the membranes that surround the central nervous system, and the sacrum.

Faye Zama is an extraordinary cranial sacral practitioner and massage therapist. Faye's discovery of massage began at age 19 and she started her practice six years later in 1984. Faye attended early Upledger cranial training at a naturopathic college in 1994. In 1999 Faye began a ten-year study of biodynamic cranial sacral work with Beth Cachet, a northwest cranial sacral educator who teaches an extensive program she developed called *Cranial Rhythms*. Beth is a member of the Northwest Cranial Sacral Therapy Association and Faye serves on the board as president as well as senior staff assisting in Cranial Rhythms trainings.

Damanhur

Damanhur, Italy, the most dynamic, successful, intentional community in the world, internationally known for their artistic, spiritual, social, educational, ecological, technological, and healing research.

Dan & Rio Watson, our dynamic duo Damanhurian guides from Ashville, North Carolina. Dan Watson, PhD psychologist, and Rio Watson, a Science of Mind practitioner, are international energy healing workshop instructors and integrative healthcare researchers of energy medicine and spiritual psychology. They are founding members and the co-directors of the LaHo-Chi Institute, an international center for spiritual energy trainings and seminars, providing continuing education units for massage therapists and bodyworkers. Dan and Rio teach throughout the United States and Europe and lead retreats to Damanhur, Italy.

Rio, wide-awake and conscious, peacefully left her body the winter of 2008. She has been a great light and amazing healer in service to this planet. We miss her and can feel her loving presence, as we know she is continuing her light journey.

Emotional Freedom Technique (EFT)

EFT is an emotional version of acupuncture wherein we stimulate certain meridian points by tapping on them with our fingertips. This addresses a new cause for emotional issues (unbalanced energy meridians). Properly done, this frequently reduces the therapeutic process from months or years down to hours or minutes. And, since emotional stress can contribute to pain, disease, and physical ailments, we often find that EFT provides astonishing physical relief.

Verna Hopkins is an exemplary massage therapist and concentrates on the pain and imbalances of the muscles and what emotions may be causing the disruption. She has used EFT with her clients and presently runs *Weighing Well* workshops for weight maintenance. She has lost 40 pounds and has kept it off since 2004 without dieting or exercise using energy exercises and EFT *tapping*.

EPFX / SCIO Quantum-Biofeedback

The SCIO Quantum Biofeedback System, now entering the third decade of its development journey, and leading the field of Bio-Energetic and Bio-Response measurement, is the accepted standard for the application of Quantum Biofeedback.

The SCIO Quantum Biofeedback System, the latest and most up-to-date technology, takes a multitude of different stress reduction programs, methods, and techniques, and merges them into a more simple—best overall—well-rounded approach. Quantum Biofeedback, working through 16 different electrical factors of the body, calculates combinations of impedance, amperage, voltage, capacitance, inductance, and resistance for Electro-Physiological Reactivity (The Xrroid Process). The body is indeed electric; therefore reactivity in the body can be measured electrically.

E-P Reactivity results are based upon the ability to establish a Tri-Vector connection for an energetic three-dimensional view of the client's current reactions to over 10,000 different items. All accomplished completely independent of user influence to help avoid bias or error. The picture painted by the reactions may help to create a better understanding of the individual factors pertinent to lifestyle and wellness. Once established, the Quantum Biofeedback auto-focus program, designed to monitor a client's reactions, helps optimize the quality and quantity of the stress reduction results.

The techniques and methods of Quantum Biofeedback stress reduction include addressing areas those most typically affected by the stressors of everyday living. Some examples of these methods and areas are the tri-vector, auto-meridian, auto-frequency, auto-color, auto-spinal, chakra, and brain wave pattern relaxation.

The SCIO Device is connected to the client via a head strap, and wrist and ankle bands. SCIO devices are being used worldwide by doctors, kinesiologists, dentists, veterinarians, naturopaths, chiropractors, homoeopaths, acupuncturists, nutritionists, psychologists, hypnotherapists, massage therapists, and many other professional practitioners.

Teresa Peers has trained extensively with the top international professionals in the field of quantum biofeedback since 2003. She sponsors Quantum Alliance head trainers and mentors students in her area of Washington state to use the EPFX effectively. In her private practice she has helped many clients reduce the stress that causes illness as well as reach optimal health.

WWW.ITSNOTWEIRDANYMORE.COM

Rochelle Clark LMP has been practicing massage therapy since 1999. She approaches her work with a sincere passion, sensitivity, and compassion. She believes that the body, mind, and spirit are divinely connected, always desiring to move toward healing and balance—and she enjoys bringing awareness and helping to facilitate that journey for each client. Rochelle is a certified Quantum Biofeedback Specialist and has been incorporating biofeedback into her practice since 2007. Rochelle enjoys using Quantum Biofeedback to help empower clients to make healthy choices and effectively reduce stressors in their lives that, over time, may interfere with optimal health and wellness. Quantum Biofeedback is an effective way to improve vitality and quality of life by focusing on pain management and stress reduction. Ralph Waldo Emerson asserted, "The first wealth is health." And in today's world of increased stresses and growing demands, maintaining one's sense of well-being is absolutely priceless.

Laura's note: Teresa and Rochelle have been of tremendous assistance for my injuries and recovery.

Etheric Spiritual Healing

Brent Howard is a bit of a prankster and an adorable child at heart. He is likely to be cracking a joke, goofing off, or conversing with a tree when you first meet him. You might even wonder if he's crazy. Don't be fooled by appearances. Brent is one of the most connected healers working today and his results prove it. Because of his exceptionally open channel to Spirit, Brent has been facilitating amazing healings for more than 20 years.

While he works with just about any issue—from eating disorders to depression to infertility—Brent's specialty at the moment is helping those with paralysis regain their freedom…a subject that hits close to home for him.

In 2001 he fell three stories off a building and broke his back and neck. He lost his ability to walk, to earn a living, even to go to the bathroom on his own. All of his *identities* were stripped away in a single moment. All that was left for him was his relationship with God.

Brent was told he was never going to walk again by allopathic doctors. That wasn't a sentence he was willing to accept so he spent a year "walking his talk" as a healer. Within nine months, he regained full function in his body. Today he even races canoes on the open ocean.

Whatever limits people are experiencing in their reality, they are unreal in *The Reality*. We are loved and supported in limitless ways by God and Brent feels it's his job to blow out the boundaries that influence us into thinking we're less than who we are.

Brent's healing work brings together a lifetime of continued study—modalities ranging from energy work to NLP—but Brent's touch goes way beyond classroom

training. He has the ability to facilitate a very clear channel to Spirit that goes beyond anything you've ever experienced on the earthly plane.

"The greatest service we can do on this planet is to remind another person of their true nature," he says.

Brent works privately. He also leads trainings where he can teach in a few hours, entire bodies of knowledge that would otherwise take years of study.

Feng Shui

Feng Shui is an ancient art and science developed over 3,000 years ago in China. It is a complex body of knowledge that reveals how to balance the energies of any given space to assure the health and good fortune for people inhabiting it.

Feng shui is based on the Taoist vision and understanding of nature, particularly on the idea that the land is alive and filled with Chi, or energy. The ancient Chinese believed that the land's energy could either make or break the kingdom, so to speak. The theories of yin and yang, as well as the five feng shui elements (earth, air, fire, water, and metal), are some of the basic aspects of a feng shui analysis that come from Taoism.

The main tools used in a feng shui analysis are the *Compass* and the *Ba-Gua*. The *Ba-Gua* is an octagonal grid containing the symbols of the *I Ching*, the ancient oracle on which feng shui is based. Knowing the *Bagua* of your home will help you understand the connection of specific feng shui areas of your home to specific areas of your life.

Cynthia Chomos is a feng shui consultant, color designer, and speaker who specializes in creating home and work environments that nurture body, mind, and spirit. Over the past decade she has provided over 2,500 consultations and appeared on TV, radio, print, and as a featured speaker at the International Feng Shui Conference and other conferences throughout the Pacific Northwest. Cynthia is the founder of the Feng Shui School for Real Estate Sales and provides home and business consultations, classes, feng shui products, and a free quarterly ezine, *Harmonious Living*.

Health Freedom

The Natural Solutions Foundation (NSF) is a non-profit corporation devoted to protecting and promoting health freedom for all Americans.

We have no other reason to exist except to support health freedom here in America and around the world. We have no commercial interests and no conflict of interest in what we do of any sort.

We know that alone we cannot safeguard our health freedoms. Therefore, the Natural Solutions Foundation is a *network of networks* created to disseminate the facts, challenges, and triumphs in our shared battle to protect, preserve, and defend our right to make our own health choices based on what we, not the government, believe are the best choices for ourselves.

History

The Natural Solutions Foundation was created to protect, promote, and defend health freedom when Rima E. Laibow, MD and Major General Albert N. Stubblebine III (US Army, Ret.) took stock of the dismal state of health freedom in the United States.

Domestically, the US faces threats such as privacy violations (HIPPA, Real ID, etc.) continuing assaults on DSHEA, witch hunts against advanced medical practitioners, stifled new medical technologies, "practice guidelines" designed to straight-jacket doctors and force them into pharmaceutical treatment of diseases and conditions that are better treated in other ways. Internationally, we face Codex Alimentarius. Domestically, we face harmonization with Codex if DSHEA and other protective laws are overturned or gutted.

General Stubblebine and Dr. Laibow looked at the current legislative climate and health-focused personnel and their stance on health and health freedom and then counted up the votes needed in the 109th Congress to push back the deadly incursions being made by Codex Alimentarius and domestic health freedom threats. They felt they had no moral and ethical choice but to close their successful full-time medical practice of natural and nutritional pharmaceutical-free advanced medicine so that they could tend to the body politic, which was sick and suffering.

Rima E. Laibow, MD is a graduate of Albert Einstein College of Medicine (1970) who believes passionately in the right of Americans to choose their own health paths. She has practiced drug-free, natural medicine for 35 years by seeking the underlying cause of every illness and ailment and treating that root cause.

She believes in using nutrients and other natural options to find, define, and treat the problems that underlie degenerative, chronic diseases and poor aging while supporting the immune and other crucial systems. She has enjoyed remarkable success with a wide assortment of cataclysmic problems.

Dr. Laibow is the president of the NeuroTherapy Certification Board, which she helped establish, in order to strengthen and develop the field of neuro-biofeedback and bring it into widespread use as a powerful, nontoxic tool for modern medicine.

Because of Dr. Laibow's awareness of the powerful, natural, nontoxic options available to treat the underlying cause of disease, she is focused on maintaining these choices for all Americans. Based on her understanding of the impact of poor nutrition and chemical/pesticide toxicity on the declining health of America, Dr. Laibow is determined to help Americans maintain the choices that allow them to protect themselves from disease and toxic harm.

Major General Albert (Bert) N. Stubblebine III (US Army, Retired)

Bert is a graduate of the US Military Academy (West Point, class of 52) who enjoyed a distinguished 32-year career in the US Army during which he commanded soldiers at every level. After his retirement he served as the VP for Intelligence Systems with BDM, a major defense contractor. He has taken this set of experiences and become involved in leading-edge medical research and development in collaboration with his wife, Rima E. Laibow, MD.

He is a long-term way-out-of-the-box thinker who redesigned the US Army's Intelligence architecture while serving as the commanding general of the US Army's Intelligence School and Center and helped to define the requirements of the US Army for future conflict. The redesign earned his place in the Intelligence Hall of Fame.

Having defended his country for 32 years and having then worked for the remainder of his career to build better ways of being and becoming well, Bert is determined not to let the forces that are threatening Americans' health freedoms prevail.

Heart Institute

The founders of *HEART* are Sheila and Gary Hay and the friends who trained Peter how to heal me with essential oils. Their vision for the *HEART* Institute is to bring the passion they have for practicing a wide spectrum of healing arts modalities to all members of humanity through teaching and hands-on practice. They wish to address all aspects of the Hue-Man Be-Ing; spiritual, emotional, and physical.

It is the HEART Institute's mission to help each soul find a path to enlighten, educate, and energize their highest self, expanding their experience and consciousness.

HEART will move toward achieving this mission by offering individual and group workshops in Alaska and across North America, online classes, and an annual retreat at the HEART Institute in the beautiful and pristine wilderness of Tok, Alaska, part of the Crown Chakra of the Earth.

Sheila and Gary Hay are the owners of Aura Borealis Wellness & Massage in Tok, Alaska. Gary and Sheila's journey into alternative healing methods began in 1997 when they became Reiki masters together. In 1998, they sold three McDonald's restaurants and moved from Anchorage, Alaska to the tiny interior town of Tok (toke), Alaska.

Sheila became a certified reflexologist through the Ontario College of Reflexology. Gary has been studying and practicing Quantum Touch Healing.

Both Gary and Sheila are certified instructors for CARE, the Center for Aromatherapy Research and Education, and teach classes nationwide on the history and use of essential oils, focusing on Raindrop Technique.

Sheila trained as a massage apprentice under Monica Molinar, LMT, and owner of Healthy Connections Wellness Center in Fairbanks, where you can attend various courses that they both teach. Her newest passion in modalities is Cranial Sacral therapy developed by Dr. John Upledger, Osteopathic MD. She is a member of the American Cranial Sacral Therapy Association and also the International Association of Health Care Practitioners, IAHP.

Gary and Sheila use their intuitive healing gifts for all of their clients, who can choose from these uplifting modalities: Cranial Sacral therapy, Reiki, massage, Raindrop Technique, Quantum Touch, reflexology, essential oil use and application, and Crystal Vibration Technique (a technique Sheila has used for the past three years).

Holy Grail Vortex Activation

Please Note: This exercise should be done with the statement, *With no harm to anyone*. Intent of exercise to be done should be stated before the exercise starts.

Bring energy to the Earth, downward direction:

First create a counter clockwise vortex in the center and visualize the downward energy penetrating the top of the apex of a tiny pyramid in the center and say:

From the point of light within the Mind of God, let Light stream forth into the minds of Humans. Let Light descend on Earth.

Create second counter clockwise vortex–three feet out–and say:

From the point of Love within the Heart of God, let Love stream forth into the hearts of Humans. May Christ return to Earth.

While these two vortexes are spinning, visualize the energy coming up in the cup of the Holy Grail.

Now reverse the flow of energy and return it in an upward direction. Spin clockwise energy field six feet out and say:

From the Center where the will of God is known, let purpose guide the wills of Humans, the purpose which the Masters know and serve.

LAURA LEGERE

(Sends the energy to the cities of Light in the fourth Dimension.)

Now spin clockwise energy field 12 feet out and say:

From the Center which we call the race of Humans, let the Plan of
Love and Light work out, and may it seal the door where evil dwells.
(Sends the energy now past the sun to the Center of the Pleiades,
which is the galaxy where Earth resides.)

Let Light and Love and Power restore the Plan of Earth.

Please Note: Be sure you have permission from Mother Earth and Divine Creator to perform this ritual. Also, it should not be done unless you have three people or you can call forth your spirit guides, guardians, and ascended masters to fill the spots to assist you if three physical beings are not available. Three people create a note of harmony. It is important that these rules be followed.

Rev. Mary Hardy is a writer, teacher, herbalist, and servant in the process of bringing a new consciousness to the planet. She has a PhD in homeopathy from the Missouri College of Naturopathic Physicians, and a BA in education from Western Michigan University. She has written two books, *The Alchemist's Handbook to Homeopathy*, and *Pyramid Energy: The Philosophy of God, The Science of Man.*

Her interest in pyramids was inspired by an incident in 1968. Mary, her husband, Dean, and their two sons, Mark and John, experienced a time loss of three to four hours. During this time, they met with the White Brotherhood and were advised to build a pyramid in their backyard. At this time they were programmed with information to bring about the healing of the planet. The whole family has access to communication with the Brotherhood. After building the large pyramid in 1975, Mary realized the importance of preparing oneself for the new consciousness that is approaching the earth. She has been advised and taught by a special teacher, John the Beloved. He is teaching her the methods of preparing oneself for advancement into the higher planes of consciousness. Mary also has memories of being trained in the mystery schools of Egypt, and other ancient initiations, in past lives.

Ho'oponopono

By Dr. Joe Vitale Sat Jul 22, 2006

Two years ago, I heard about a therapist in Hawaii who cured an entire ward of criminally insane patients—without ever seeing any of them. The psychologist would study an inmate's chart and then look within himself to see how he created that person's illness. As he improved himself, the patient improved.

When I first heard this story, I thought it was an urban legend. How could anyone heal anyone else by healing himself? How could even the best self-improvement master cure the criminally insane? It didn't make any sense. It wasn't logical, so I dismissed the story.

However, I heard it again a year later. I heard that the therapist had used a Hawaiian healing process called Ho'oponopono. I had never heard of it, yet I couldn't let it leave my mind. If the story was at all true, I had to know more. I had always understood "total responsibility" to mean that I am responsible for what I think and do. Beyond that, it's out of my hands. I think that most people think of total responsibility that way. We're responsible for what we do, not what anyone else does—but that's wrong.

The Hawaiian therapist who healed those mentally ill people would teach me an advanced new perspective about total responsibility. His name is Dr. Ihaleakala Hew Len. We probably spent an hour talking on our first phone call. I asked him to tell me the complete story of his work as a therapist. He explained that he worked at Hawaii State Hospital for four years. That ward where they kept the criminally insane was dangerous.

Psychologists quit on a monthly basis. The staff called in sick a lot or simply quit. People would walk through that ward with their backs against the wall, afraid of being attacked by patients. It was not a pleasant place to live, work, or visit.

Dr. Len told me that he never saw patients. He agreed to have an office and to review their files. While he looked at those files, he would work on himself. As he worked on himself, patients began to heal.

After a few months, patients who had to be shackled were being allowed to walk freely, he told me. Others who had to be heavily medicated were getting off their medications. And those who had no chance of ever being released were being freed. I was in awe. Not only that, he went on, but the staff began to enjoy coming to work. Absenteeism and turnover disappeared. We ended up with more staff than we needed because patients were being released, and all the staff was showing up to work. Today, that ward is closed.

This is where I had to ask the million-dollar question: What were you doing within yourself that caused those people to change? I was simply healing the part of me that created them, he said. I didn't understand. Dr. Len explained that total responsibility for your life means that everything in your life—simply because it is in your life—is your responsibility. In a literal sense the entire world is your creation.

Whew. This is tough to swallow. Being responsible for what I say or do is one thing. Being responsible for what everyone in my life says or does is quite another. Yet, the truth is this: if you take complete responsibility for your life, then everything you see, hear, taste, touch, or in any way experience is your responsibility because it is in your life. This means that terrorist activity, the president, the economy or anything you experience and don't like is up for you to heal. They don't exist, in a manner of speaking, except as projections from inside you. The problem isn't with them, it's with you, and to change them, you have to change you.

I know this is tough to grasp, let alone accept or actually live. Blame is far easier than total responsibility, but as I spoke with Dr. Len, I began to realize that healing for him and in Ho'oponopono means loving yourself. If you want to improve your life, you have to heal your life. If you want to cure anyone, even a mentally ill criminal, you do it by healing you.

I asked Dr. Len how he went about healing himself. What was he doing, exactly, when he looked at those patients' files?

I just kept saying,

"I'm sorry" and "I love you" over and over again, he explained.

"That's it?"

"That's it."

Turns out that loving yourself is the greatest way to improve yourself, and as you improve yourself, you improve your world.

Let me give you a quick example of how this works: one day, someone sent me an email that upset me. In the past I would have handled it by working on my emotional hot buttons or by trying to reason with the person who sent the nasty message. This time, I decided to try Dr. Len's method. I kept silently saying,

"I'm sorry" and "I love you."

I didn't say it to anyone in particular. I was simply evoking the spirit of love to heal within me what was creating the outer circumstance. Within an hour I got an email from the same person. He apologized for his previous message. Keep in mind that I didn't take any outward action to get that apology. I didn't even write him back. Yet, by saying, "I love you," I somehow healed within me what was creating him. I later attended a

Ho'oponopono workshop run by Dr. Len. He's now 70 years old, considered a grandfatherly shaman, and is somewhat reclusive.

He praised my book, *The Attractor Factor*. He told me that as I improve myself, my book's vibration will raise, and everyone will feel it when they read it. In short, as I improve, my readers will improve.

"What about the books that are already sold and out there?" I asked.

"They aren't out there," he explained, once again blowing my mind with his mystic wisdom.

"They are still in you."

In short, there is no out there. It would take a whole book to explain this advanced technique with the depth it deserves. Suffice it to say that whenever you want to improve anything in your life, there's only one place to look: inside you. When you look, do it with love.

Ho'oponopono is a cleansing method that gets you to the *Zero State*. In Hawaiian: Hoo means *cause* and ponopono means *perfection*. Ho'oponopono is the ancient Hawaiian healing method that heals and transmutes/cleans all energies with current and past situations and people, all the way down the ancestory lines, yours and others throughout the *entire* Universe. All you need to do is say the four key phrases: (1) I'm so sorry (2) Please forgive me (3) I love you (4) Thank you. At first you might not feel a thing. It matters not, the work is still being done. Eventually, you really *will* feel a difference in yourself and in others around you. You will have cleansed your life, continuing to cleanse, and brought yourself into a better frame of mind, body *and* soul!

Dr. Joe Vitale. According to *Succeed* magazine, Dr. Joe *Mr. Fire* Vitale is one of the five top marketing specialists in the world today and is known to his readers, customers, and seminar attendees as the world's first hypnotic writer. He is the author of the international #1 best-seller, *The Attractor Factor*, the #1 best-seller *Life's Missing Instruction Manual*, the #1 best-selling e-book *Hypnotic Writing*, and the #1 best-selling *Nightingale-Conant* audio program, *The Power of Outrageous Marketing*, among numerous other works. *Zerolimits* is one of his newer books and is about Ho'oponopono and a fantastic beginning that encourages you to attend Dr. Hew Len's Ho'oponopono workshop. I loved the book and the workshop and use the material constantly. Dr. Vitale is also one of the stars of the hit movie *The Secret*. Joe is a certified hypnotherapist, a certified metaphysical practitioner, a certified Chi Kung healer, and an ordained minister. He holds a doctorate degree in metaphysical science and another doctorate degree in marketing and is a proud member of the National Speakers Association.

Morrnah Nalamaku Simeona, Creator of Self Identity through Ho'oponopono (SITH) (1913 – 1992) Morrnah Nalamaku Simeona, a native Hawaiian Kahuna Lapa'au, is the creator of Self Identity through Ho'oponopono (SITH). As the Master Teacher, she lectured and conducted SITH classes around the world, including at medical facilities, colleges and universities. Morrnah gave SITH classes at the United Nations three times. The Hongwanji Mission of Honolulu and the Hawaii State Legislature honored Morrnah for her work and expertise in the Hawaiian language and culture by naming her a *Living Treasure of Hawaii* in 1983.

Ihaleakala Hew Len, Ph.D., Master Teacher of SITH (1982 – Present) Dr. Hew Len has extensive experiences working with the developmentally disabled and the criminally mentally ill and their families. Self Identity through Ho'oponopono (SITH) is central to his work as an educator. He has been conducting SITH classes around the world for over twenty years.

Kabbalah

The **Universal Kabbalah**, meaning, *to receive* or *that which is received*, serves as a simple system of understanding yourself and reconnecting to the divine spirit and divine essence within. Passed down through the ancient mystical traditions yet independent from any specific religion, it helps you answer all the important questions that you need to ask in life, and it acts as the most powerful tool on the planet for manifestation, self-discovery, and empowerment. Through the Kabbalah you come to *Know Thyself* more fully, the gates of the soul open up, the true self becomes revealed, and the inner lights of hope, passion, and inspiration come alive. You can learn about this powerful tool and how it can enhance your life through the Mystery School in this resource directory.

Lymphatic Drainage

Lymphatic Drainage therapy consists of a manual massage, performed by a lymphatic drainage therapist. A lymphatic drainage massage primarily focuses on specific lymph nodes and points of the body, as well as the natural flow of the lymphatic system. Proponents of lymphatic drainage believe that the process will reduce blockages of the lymphatic system, which in turn promotes a healthier body. When the lymphatic system becomes blocked, lymph nodes may become swollen. Further, the system fails to remove the body's toxins and can even affect white blood cell counts. Lymphatic drainage is believed to reduce blockage, which promotes health in the lymphatic system as well as other bodily systems such as the circulatory, respiratory, muscular, and endocrine systems. Some therapists believe that lymphatic drainage therapy can also reduce allergies, menstrual cramps, colds, and other viruses.

Rochelle Clark, LMP, has been in private practice since 1999. She is continually seeking to expand her professional education for the benefit of her clients and began studying lymphatic drainage massage in 2003. Rochelle took her education in lymphatic drainage to a deeper level by becoming formally certified in this delicate work. Rochelle says lymphatic drainage is easy on the body, yet the effects for her clients are deeply profound. Due to the gentle nature of lymphatic work, Rochelle frequently works with acute injuries and pre- and post- surgery clients (with doctor permission). She believes that the body, mind, and spirit are divinely connected, always desiring to move toward healing and balance as she enjoys bringing awareness of that journey for each client.

Medical Intuition & Food Allergies

Caroline Sutherland, Medical Intuitive

The key to medical intuition or any other intuitive ability is a quiet, receptive mind. The rational or trained mind becomes the filter through which the intuitive impressions are received. Meditation, prayer, and quiet receptivity are prerequisites for this ability. Medical intuition comes from the spiritual level; where everything is known.

While the emotions and the spiritual are taken into account, Caroline's strength seems to lie specifically on the physical level, as a result of her training in environmental medicine, where she worked as an allergy-testing technician for many years. This gift came to her suddenly when she was a physician's assistant and allergy-testing technician in a busy clinic devoted to environmental medicine. Caroline had been trained in the use of highly specialized allergy testing equipment. She began to hear a very distinct inner voice guiding her to areas of the body and specific substances to test, which were not ordered on the test forms. She shared the information that she was hearing with the physician and because he was an open-minded individual, he agreed to evaluate its validity. Then in a very short time, because of the finely tuned results, people were getting well and the clinic had a yearlong waiting list.

As soon as Caroline connected with the person she received a flood of information. She can perceive all the foods to which a person may be sensitive or allergic, environmental factors, key systems that may be out of balance, hormones, the GI tract, immunity, weight problems, etc. as well as underlying causes and when they may have begun and what precipitated them.

The information is very specific. The imbalances are only part of the picture. Perceptions regarding *correction* or what may be needed to bring the body back into balance in terms of diet, supplements, botanicals, homeopathy, lifestyle changes, and associated modalities are also given to her. Among other things, Caroline has a sense of timing—how long it will take the person to rebalance, their level of compliance or if indeed they are likely to recover.

In 1999 through a fortuitous meeting, Caroline's career took an important turn. Louise Hay, founder of Hay House publishing in California, was attracted to her work both as a client and a student. In the fall of 2001, *The Body Knows–How to tune in to your body and improve your health,* was published and her career has escalated since then.

Miracle Mineral Supplement

From Laura:

I have been introduced to a simple, inexpensive way that may help rid the body of parasites, candida, fungus, and disease.

The inventor/scientist who discovered it does not live in this country and the medical cartel along with the World Health Organization are not interested in his simple, inexpensive, fast cure. This man is working with the African government and is experiencing a 100% cure rate of malaria and AIDS. Malaria may be rid of in a matter of hours.

He has discovered an inexpensive substance called sodium chlorite. When activated with citric acid for three minutes, sodium chlorite becomes an amazing immune system booster and can help rid the body of parasites, candida, fungus, and disease. He calls it the Miracle Mineral Supplement and ironically his name is Jim Humble. There are many testimonials of people having cured themselves of Hep A, B, and C, cancer, etc. I have used it as a cleanser and dropped back to a maintenance dose. Peter has practically rid his body of Hep C and his liver is repaired according to his blood tests, along with much more energy than he has felt in years as well as clear urine. Peter was exposed to a lot of chemicals working for the phone company for 30 years and MMS may have been one of the natural substances that helped neutralize the poisons. The chemicals in his body made it easy for the Hep C to thrive. Not to mention all the mercury from his old fillings. The fillings have been removed and detoxing from mercury is not fun; chelex from Young Living helped with that. Peter peeled off his health issues in layers with natural remedies and was happy to discover one substance that can help so many issues. I noticed my sugar cravings subsided after three days, which is an indication that candida is resolving for me. A maintenance dose may keep it away, along with parasites and fungus.

One bottle of Miracle Mineral Supplement is $20 and lasts a whole family for one year. I recommend ordering Jim's book Breakthrough (The Miracle Mineral Supplement of the 21st Century) as well. Much of the money goes to supporting his African project of curing malaria and AIDS.

I believe it benefits many of us to keep it on hand, do a cleanse with it, and then keep up a maintenance routine on it. MMS is not for everyone and it is up to you to decide with help from a medical professional you trust.

Be careful not to overdo it and detox too fast. Detoxing with MMS may be really uncomfortable. You might experience diarrhea and nausea at first as toxins leave your body, but you can regulate the amount and back off if you prefer not to have nausea. The diarrhea is okay temporarily, as it should clear up anyway after the major part of the detox. Peter did not experience diarrhea so much as just dumping a lot; I did a little. Jim recommends starting out with two drops of MMS and ten drops of the citric acid twice a day. For every drop of MMS he recommends five drops of 10% citric acid solution. Lemon juice, vinegar, or citric acid crystals dissolved in distilled water are preferred. Citric acid crystals can be purchased on the website or at most health food stores. If you have a serious illness, you may want to start out with two drops twice a day and work your way up to 15 drops three times a day according to Jim's book. Bedtime is a good time to take a dose as it may make you sleepy. Please study the information on the website and buy Jim's book.

Jim Humble discovered a simple health drink cure for malaria in South America during a prospecting venture. When he returned from the prospecting trip he worked on the health drink formula for several years, sending it to friends in Africa who were able to use it in the field. Eventually a missionary group invited him to Africa, where he personally treated over 2,000 malaria victims and those he trained while there treated over 75,000 malaria cases.

The formula was a simple health drink that had already been used for years for other reasons. Jim drastically improved the effectiveness by adding a few drops of vinegar to the drink. Since that time thousands of cases of many different diseases have been treated with complete success.

Before and during the time Jim was doing his work in the Missions in Africa thousands of clinical trials were being conducted in hospitals and clinics throughout the world using essentially the same formula that Jim used. More than a hundred thousand clinical trials over a period of 15 years verified the effectiveness of Jim's treatment and success in Africa.

The difference is that while thousands of trials and treatments were conducted in hospitals throughout the world the data was never really brought forward for public consumption.

Jim, on the other hand, brought the treatment to the world. His book not only gives complete details of his work, but it also has a chapter, written by Dr. Hesselink, listing over 160 scientific papers describing more than 100,000 scientific tests using essentially the same formula that Jim used and still uses. These tests verify all of Jim's basic concepts covering mostly data concerning malaria.

Jim started his career in the aerospace industry, where he quickly became a research engineer. He worked on the first intercontinental missile, the moon vehicle, wrote instruction manuals for the first vacuum tube computers, set up experiments for A-bomb explosions, worked on secret radio control electronics, set up experiments in electrical generation by magneto hydro dynamics, complete wired the first machine to be controlled by computers at Hughes aircraft company, and invented the first automatic garage door opener.

In the mining field he wrote four books updating older technology and improving the health hazards for those involved. He first overcame the hazards of mercury and invented ways of eliminating mercury from mining altogether. His technology included methods of eliminating chemical leaching, finally using nothing but water for the recovery of gold.

Jim's immediate goal is to return to Africa to eliminate all of the malaria in a single African nation in order to prove to the world that it is possible.

Mystery School

Since ancient times, Mystery Schools have existed across the globe for those who feel called to walk a life path of true knowledge, understanding, and wisdom that integrates the seen and unseen worlds. Mystery school teachings inspire the soul, train the mind, and hand down tools of empowerment that can be applied toward practical success and fulfillment in life. Traditionally, mystery school teachings have helped people gain understanding, develop wisdom, and strengthen inner guidance. The training they offer helps to clear limiting physical energies and enhance spiritual direction toward a more purposeful existence. They have been likened to universities for the soul, where the curriculum focuses on how to awaken and develop our highest potential, and to attain divine awareness. Beyond merely teaching, the mystery schools help students to refine conscious potential, build focus, and activate the innate powers through a series of initiations, ceremonies, and sacred meditations. The purpose of the Mystery Tradition is the conscious realization of one's true self and one's connection to others, both physical and spiritual. With this expanded awareness comes the power to bridge spiritual energies into the physical world for healing and transformation, at a personal and planetary level.

Rocky Mountain International

The Rocky Mountain Mystery School, in the lineage of King Salomon, has direct contact with the Hierarchy of Light and draws upon the powers of Heaven and the Universe. We conduct teachings of the great mysteries and the old magick of the ages. The Mystery School does not represent any religion or political ideas but is solely interested in the powers that build up our lives in a positive way.

All true seekers of spiritual life are invited to partake of the revealing of the Great Mysteries of Life. We see all things in an eternal perspective and we accept all humans equally without prejudices toward any race, color, or circumstances. Our teachers travel all over the world to bring these teachings to all who seek them.

Gudni Gudnason: After studying with the Hermetic Order of the Golden Dawn in England for several years, Gudni was sent out into the world to teach. He has trained in many other mystery schools in places such as Tibet, Africa, Transylvania, and Japan and has had initiations in many different mysteries such as the Celtic, the Norse, and the Egyptian.

Gudni moved to America in 1995 to found the Rocky Mountain Mystery School in North America. He has worked rigorously on spreading the mystery school tradition and has centers in the United States, Japan, Canada, Philippines, India, England, France, South Africa, Ireland, China, Taiwan, Australia, Iceland, and Sweden.

Gudni has been teaching the Kaballah since 1976 and was trained first by a rabbi in the traditional Jewish Kaballah and later in Universal Kaballah by the original Order of the Golden Dawn.

Gudni has a doctoral degree in metaphysics and a degree in psychology. He won the Swedish Artist of the Year Award, Poet of the Year and Businessman of the Year. He has been awarded The International Peace Prize for Humanitarian Work from the United Cultural World Society. He is a master teacher and welcomes anyone who desires this knowledge.

Crystal Temple (Mystery School affiliate in Portland, OR)

Our goal for Crystal Temple is to provide a supportive environment for accessing our holistic nature. As people do this they empower themselves in all aspects of their life! At this time on Earth, a rapid evolution is taking place from within mankind. This can be devastating to those who are blindsided by the huge changes taking place. We offer the tools, training, and group support to put people in control of their growth and not be victim to it. The path we offer draws support from the many beings on the spiritual realms. The work we do at the Temple addresses body, mind, and spirit in a holistic fashion. Many are stepping forward to empower themselves in these times of change.

David Recht, Director. David was born in Berkley, California, grew up in the bay area and moved to Oregon pursuing an engineering degree and eventually settled in Portland. After spending the bulk of the last 20 years studying metaphysics, alternative healing and free energy, he began his formal training within the Ancient Mystery Schools in the Spring of 2003. Through these years of persistent study, David has mastered many types of esoteric energy work and now finds himself deep into 'the doing' of the work. After dreaming of the Crystal Temple for the past 20 years it has grown, evolved and gradually precipitated into the physical. It has taken dedication, sacrifice and persistence to bring forth this wonderful light center into the world and truly feeds his heart to bring support to those who walk through the doors of this space.

Amanda Jones, Assistant Director. Amanda was born in Portland and grew up in rural Eastern Oregon. A natural athlete, she swam competitively for 15 years and still currently holds four records. She also excelled in volleyball and secured an athletic scholarship that helped finance bachelor's degrees in business, history, sociology, and anthropology. She pursued a career in business and finance, successfully owning, operating, and selling two businesses, and after ten successful years in the corporate structure, she became discontented and unfulfilled. As a small girl, her natural sixth sense abilities were *turned on* and over time and study eventually she learned how to regulate them in order to *fit in*. In 2001 she began formal training and started studying with a Choctaw medicine man and continued that study, learning the Native American arts of communing with Spirit. This quickly became a passion in her life, and as she continued her search for more knowledge and empowerments, including apprenticing with a Wiccan Priestess, learning to weave the magickal arts into everyday life. Feeling like there was a piece that was missing, in the fall of

2004, she began formal initiatory training with one of the seven Ancient Mystery Schools, the Rocky Mountain Mystery School, and those missing pieces started to fall into place.

Lifestream, Inc. is a non-profit Learning Center and Mystery School affiliate in Roanoke, VA, offering classes, workshops, and programs that give people opportunities to practice well-being, inner personal work, and take responsibility for their own health and well-being. Scholarships are available for their programs.

The Lifestream Learning Annex houses practitioners seeing clients, classes, lectures, workshops, and a bookstore featuring 20% off books and music. A fine selection of health products are also available.

Organic Locally Grown Produce in Washington State

Full Circle Farm is a 300-acre certified organic produce farm in Carnation, Washington. Full Circle Farm cultivates over 125 varieties of fruits, vegetables, and herbs, using sustainable farming practices that focus on soil health as the foundation for nutritious organic produce.

Their top quality produce is available through their year-round CSA (Community Supported Agriculture) Program and found in local farmers markets, restaurants, and grocery stores. Members of the CSA Program have the ability to customize box contents and have the option of ordering from Full Circle's *Green Grocer,* which offers a variety of products that can be delivered with their box. Choose from organic fair-trade chocolate and coffee, fresh eggs from free-roaming organic chickens, and other seasonally available fruits and vegetables.

Laura's note: I recommend that wherever you live it benefits everyone to support they're local organic sustainable farms. This practice keeps your body, the local economy, and the environment healthier.

Politics –Ron Paul, Revolution, Ethics, Education, and Participation

Congressman Ron Paul is the leading advocate for freedom in our nation's capital. As a member of the US House of Representatives, Dr. Paul tirelessly works for limited constitutional government, low taxes, free markets, and a return to sound monetary policies. He is known among his congressional colleagues and his constituents for his consistent voting record. Dr. Paul never votes for legislation unless the proposed measure is expressly authorized by the Constitution. In the words of former Treasury Secretary William Simon, Dr. Paul is the *one exception to the Gang of 535* on Capitol Hill.

WWW.ITSNOTWEIRDANYMORE.COM

Ron Paul was born and raised in Pittsburgh, Pennsylvania. He graduated from Gettysburg College and the Duke University School of Medicine, before proudly serving as a flight surgeon in the US Air Force during the 1960s. He and his wife, Carol, moved to Texas in 1968, where he began his medical practice in Brazoria County. As a specialist in obstetrics/gynecology, Dr. Paul has delivered more than 4,000 babies. He and Carol, who reside in Lake Jackson, Texas, are the proud parents of five children and have 17 grandchildren.

While serving in Congress during the late 1970s and early 1980s, Dr. Paul's limited-government ideals were not popular in Washington. In 1976, he was one of only four Republican congressmen to endorse Ronald Reagan for president.

During that time, Congressman Paul served on the House Banking committee, where he was a strong advocate for sound monetary policy and an outspoken critic of the Federal Reserve's inflationary measures. Dr. Paul consistently voted to lower or abolish federal taxes, spending, and regulation, and used his House seat to actively promote the return of government to its proper constitutional levels. In 1984, he voluntarily relinquished his House seat and returned to his medical practice.

Dr. Paul returned to Congress in 1997 to represent the 14th congressional district of Texas. He presently serves on the House Committee on Financial Services and the House Committee on Foreign Affairs. He continues to advocate a dramatic reduction in the size of the federal government and a return to constitutional principles.

Congressman Paul's consistent voting record prompted one of his congressional colleagues to say, "Ron Paul personifies the Founding Fathers ideal of the citizen-statesman. He makes it clear that his principles will never be compromised, and they never are." Another colleague observed, "There are few people in public life who, through thick and thin, rain or shine, stick to their principles. Ron Paul is one of those few."

Brief Overview of Congressman Paul's Record:

He has never voted to raise taxes.

He has never voted for an unbalanced budget.

He has never voted for a federal restriction on gun ownership.

He has never voted to raise congressional pay.

He has never taken a government-paid junket.

He has never voted to increase the power of the executive branch.

He voted against the Patriot Act.

He voted against regulating the Internet.

He voted against the Iraq war.

He does not participate in the lucrative congressional pension program.

He returns a portion of his annual congressional office budget to the US Treasury every year.

Congressman Paul introduces numerous pieces of substantive legislation each year, probably more than any single member of Congress.

LAURA LEGERE

Laura's note: As the Political Establishment performed their normal illegal tactics to keep Dr. Paul from being a front runner, I believe his message will still influence the next administration anyway. Dr. Paul inspired us as individuals to participate and this will not die down. Read his book, The Revolution (a manifesto). It has been number one on The New York Times best seller list as well as Amazon. His latest literary masterpiece is End the Fed, a must read. There is much more we can do to change things than just going to the polls to vote. I have learned a tremendous amount since participating in the caucuses, being a delegate and applying to be a PCO (Precinct Community Officer). We can vote the Republican Hierarchy in or out as PCOs.

I attended the Washington State Republican Convention in Spokane, WA, May 29, 30th and 31st 2008 as a volunteer. I wanted to witness the process, support the Ron Paul delegates, and watch for rule violations. Although I am not versed in Washington State and Republican Party rules, I was around some who were. The old Republican guard trickster behavior was pretty obvious in spite of my being uninformed of the rules. The passionate Ron Paulers were in force and accounted for 1/3 of the convention. I heard one RP delegate stand up on the convention floor and say he had overheard a McCain supporter say he was called in by the GOP; offered expenses paid and given automatic delegate status to participate in the convention. If that is true, I wonder how many others this illegal offer was made to. It was obvious during the voting that the McCain drone delegates voted the way they were told and did not think on their own as they followed the yes and no signs waving in the air. The RP delegates brought forth many points to make things fair and were supposedly outvoted, but that was hard to tell. The temporary chair would declare we were two-thirds outvoted, but my observation along with others did not see the two-thirds majority. The biggest offense was the McCain delegates walking out so we would not have a quorum to vote on resolutions. I believe this was an example of how Congress gets nothing done. We had 67 resolutions we wanted to vote on. Some really good ones too, Repeal the Patriot Act, Reinvestigate 911, Get Rid of the Federal Reserve, Fairness in the Courts, Revoke CODEX, No Mandatory Real IDs, Internet Neutrality, etc. The head chair was a fair guy and gave us a head count to see if we may have a quorum after all. Well, we had 50 people over a quorum, and literally began singing The Star-Spangled Banner. The first resolution was presented as the McCain drones came back in to manipulate the process some more. The resolution on the floor as the McCain drones filed in but were not seated yet was, The president does not have the authority to declare war without the consent of Congress. It passed almost unanimously. I know it's already in the Constitution, but it has not been adhered to and to declare it on the Republican platform might reinforce it, most definitely our resolve. Then the McCain drones created some other way to thwart the process and we were dismissed and the convention was over.

This may very well backfire for the Republican Party. There were some ethical McCain delegates who were embarrassed by what they witnessed and did not vote the party line. The RP delegates had a lawyer observe with some well versed in the rules old RP ethical Republicans to witness violations. They found hundreds of violations and are pursuing a lawsuit. Texas has already filed. We were told that this same scenario had been taking place across the country. It's all on YouTube, see for yourself.

One Ron Paul delegate, a passionate young man, told our large RP crowd that he was approached by a McCain supporter who said he would pay his expenses to the National Convention plus an extra $500 if he would vote for McCain the first go around so as not to embarrass the Republican Party. This young RP delegate told him to shove it. The revolution is about principles and ethics, something most politicians are not accustomed to.

I have had the privilege to meet, converse, and organize with many wonderful, thoughtful, caring individuals through this process. The power of our focus and large numbers was making headway with a momentum that will continue to build.

A delightful person I have come to know named Al Shaefer was running for my 7th Congressional District. He is a very healthy, passionate 82-year-old retired physics professor with many other talents too numerous to name here. Simply put, he is a principled Ron Paul Republican, humorous, thought-provoking humanitarian and I enjoy his company immensely.

June 6th 2008: I am happy to hear that Obama is the democratic nominee and know that his administration will be influenced by us. Let's participate!

September 6th 2008: My Ron Paul delegate contacts at the Republican National Convention had tales to tell. Theirs along with all other RP delegate campaign materials were confiscated without the confiscators identifying themselves and giving a good reason for doing it. The RP delegates were closely followed everywhere because the McCain campaign was so paranoid that they would create a scene. Every time a RP delegate had the rare opportunity to approach the mic, it was conveniently turned off. This happened over and over again. Then the McCain camp gave the RP delegates a choice to either vote for McCain or leave; so much for the so-called democratic process.

Laura's update Nov 12th 2008: I notice my June 6th statement above assumes Obama won the presidency as well he did! Even though I believe the two-party system has been a sham and the Democratic and Republican parties are owned by corporations and the same corporations own both parties, something unusual happened. Coming from a spiritual, intuitive perspective Obama's win showed the world's collective consciousness wanted to make real positive changes for humanity and the planet. My inner guidance confirmed by my spiritual connections told me that Obama would prove to be a truthful, honest, ethical, dynamic leader and his positive influence would raise people's self-esteem. During the campaign, if he had addressed the same issues to the extent that Ron Paul did, he would never have been allowed by the political establishment to make it to the White House. I did vote for Obama and for the first time felt that I did not vote for the lesser of two evils and for someone who could actually win and follow through with what he promised. I felt comforted by the focus of the entire world sending America and Barack and his family positive energy. Just think about what we could heal, change, release, and create together with collective positive consciousness. I believe President-elect Barack Obama represents all ethnic nationalities as he himself stated he is a mutt and this will help mend our divided illusion. Barack inspired grassroots participation on a massive scale as did Ron Paul. My vision is for the impassioned individuals in the groundswell of the grassroots movement to have intelligent, heartfelt dialogue and create a harmonious planet that is blind to parties. Let's use ethics and gross national happiness as the measure of how we are doing. The Netherlands is a great template for ethical government; it has eight political parties, everyone has a voice, and they accomplish constructive projects for the good of the whole in a reasonable amount of time.

If the Republicans are going to make a comeback, it is imperative that they begin to welcome new people, new ideas, and start playing fair. At this time my observation is that the only way the Republicans win is low voter turnout, voter suppression, and vote fraud. Now that record numbers of voters are participating, and cheating is more closely watched, Republicans must reinvent themselves if they want a party at all.

Campaign for Liberty

CFL was created by the Ron Paul grassroots movement to help our political leaders be accountable to the Constitution and the people. To promote and defend the great American principles of individual liberty, constitutional government, sound money, free markets, and a noninterventionist foreign policy, by means of educational and political activity.

Mises Institute – Honorable Economics

It is the mission of the Mises Institute to restore a high place for theory in economics and the social sciences, encourage a revival of critical historical research, and draw attention to neglected traditions in Western philosophy. In this cause, the Mises Institute works to advance the Austrian School of economics and the Misesian tradition, and, in application, defends the market economy, private property, sound money, and peaceful international relations, while opposing government intervention as economically and socially destructive.

You can line up 100 professional war historians and political scientists to talk about the 20th century, and not one is likely to mention the role of the Fed in funding US militarism. And yet the story of central banking is one step removed from the story of atom bombs and death camps. It is the most important priority of the state to keep its money machine hidden behind a curtain. Anyone who dares pull the curtain back is accused of every manner of intellectual crime. We must end the conspiracy of silence on this issue.

Ludwig von Mises (1881-1973) by Murray N. Rothbard

"Economics deals with society's fundamental problems; it concerns everyone and belongs to all. It is the main and proper study of every citizen."

One of the most notable economists and social philosophers of the 20th century, Ludwig von Mises, in the course of a long and highly productive life, developed an integrated, deductive science of economics based on the fundamental axiom that individual human beings act purposively to achieve desired goals. Even though his economic analysis itself was *value-free*—in the sense of being irrelevant to values held by economists—Mises concluded that the only viable economic policy for the human race was a policy of unrestricted laissez-faire, of free markets, and the unhampered exercise of the right of private property, with government strictly limited to the defense of person and property within its territorial area.

For Mises was able to demonstrate (a) that the expansion of free markets, the division of labor, and private capital investment is the only possible path to the prosperity and flourishing of the human race; (b) that socialism would be disastrous for a modern economy because the absence of private ownership of land and capital goods prevents any sort of rational pricing, or estimate of costs, and (c) that government intervention, in addition to hampering and crippling the market, would prove counterproductive and cumulative, leading inevitably to socialism unless the entire issue of interventions was repealed.

Holding these views, and hewing to truth indomitably in the face of a century increasingly devoted to statism and collectivism, Mises became famous for his *intransigence* in insisting on a non-inflationary gold standard and on laissez-faire.

Effectively barred from any paid university post in Austria and later in the United States, Mises pursued his course gallantly. As the chief economic adviser to the Austrian government in the 1920s, Mises was singlehandedly able to slow down Austrian inflation; and he developed his own *private seminar*, which attracted the outstanding young economists, social scientists, and philosophers throughout Europe. As the founder of the *neo-Austrian School* of economics, Mises's business cycle theory, which blamed inflation and depressions on inflationary bank credit encouraged by central banks, was adopted by most younger economists in England in the early 1930s as the best explanation of the Great Depression.

> "If the American people ever allow private banks to control the issue of their money, first by inflation and then by deflation, the banks and corporations that will grow up around them, will deprive the people of their property until their children will wake up homeless on the continent their fathers conquered."
>
> —Thomas Jefferson

> "It is well enough that people of the nation do not understand our banking and monetary system, for if they did, I believe there

would be a revolution before tomorrow morning."
—Henry Ford

"Most Americans have no real understanding of the operations of the international moneylenders...the accounts of the Federal Reserve have never been audited. It operates outside the control of Congress and...manipulates the credit of the United States"
—Sen. Barry Goldwater (R. –AZ)

For several years there has been a $50,000 reward for anyone who can show proof of the IRS code or law that states the income tax is compulsory or mandatory. No one has collected to date.

Ron Paul has been educating the public about the truth of our economy and the Fed and as a result experienced a media blackout during his presidential campaign. The bought paid and sold their soul down the road media and the owner monopoly do not want us to know the truth about economics. Do your own research and come to your own conclusions.

Psychic Training

Psychic Awakenings provides a safe space for sensitive people to explore and develop their psychic abilities. We offer a variety of readings, psychic development classes, and a community of warm, caring people.

It is by developing your psychic abilities that helps you to find the answers to your deepest yearnings to know:

*   Who am I really underneath my busyness, my masks, and who I "think" I am?
*   What is the purpose and meaning of my life?
*   How can I reach my full potential and use it to help make the world a better place?
*   How can I create genuine, meaningful relationships with others?

As director, **Madeline Hartman's** extensive experience in both conventional and alternative counseling gives her a unique perspective and a wide range of skills with which she can support you. Since 1980 she has offered spiritual counseling in the form of readings, healings, and psychic development classes.

Her training began at the Berkeley Psychic Institute/Church of Divine Man, where she was ordained as a spiritual minister. While at Berkeley she taught meditation and healing classes for five years.

Relationship Awakening

The Three Stages of Relationship by David Deida

By understanding your current style of intimate relationship, you can understand the next step you need to take. Which of the three styles is most like your current, or recent, relationship: Dependence, 50/50, or Intimate Communion? Each of these three styles is also a stage that you can grow through, if you are willing to be lovingly humorous about your own patterns in intimacy.

1. Dependence Relationship

"Men are men and women are women."

In the imaginary video, were you are viewing a man and a woman in the abandoned throes of sexual ecstasy, or was the man subjugating, biting, and penetrating the woman against her will? In a Dependence Relationship, sex and power are often painfully mixed up; partners often confuse some version of the master/slave relationship with real love. They are engaged in some kind of power play. In a Dependence Relationship, one partner often needs to feel in control while the other partner often gives up his or her authentic power in order to feel loved and accepted. A Dependence Relationship involves partners who become dependent on each other for money, emotional support, parenting, or sex. Although the sex is sometimes good in this style of relationship (especially during the making-up period after a fight), partners often end up feeling limited by old-style gender roles or by an imbalance of financial or physical power. So they attempt to transition to the next style of relationship. To do so they learn to build personal boundaries and take care of themselves, rather than always catering to the needs of their partners.

2. 50/50 Relationship

"Safe boundaries and equal expectations for men and women."

Partners in a 50/50 Relationship want to feel safe, so the videotape might seem harsh and violent to them. On the surface, they might seem completely turned off and react as if any form of forceful and passionate sexual ravishment is an act of rape. Deep down, however, they might be wistfully turned on, reminded of the depth of sexual loving that may be missing from their safe but lukewarm love life. The 50/50 Relationship is the "modern" style of relationship that is based on two independent people coming together and working out an equitable partnership. Each partner is expected to shoulder half the responsibilities, more or less, right down the middle. Each often has their own source of income, and together they negotiate a 50/50 plan to divide household duties, parenting, and financial obligations. To accomplish this, they attempt to strike their own inner balance between Masculine and Feminine qualities, both at home and at the workplace. However, as many of us have discovered, there is a potential problem with this ideal of a 50/50 Relationship. We begin to lose our aliveness. Sexuality loses its passion. Our inner fire begins to fade. And we feel an incompleteness at our center. Why? Because many of us have a sexual essence that is naturally more Masculine or Feminine than it is equally balanced or Neutral. Thus, a side-effect of this effort toward 50/50 is the suppression or starvation of our naturally more Masculine or Feminine sexual essence. For some of us, a cooperative partnership which emphasizes communication and shared responsibilities is sufficient. Others in this situation eventually suffer a feeling of incompleteness and develop a yearning to touch and be touched far more deeply and more passionately than a 50/50 Relationship often allows.

3. Intimate Communion
   "I relax into oneness and spontaneously give my deepest gift."
   If we have grown beyond a 50/50 Relationship, we are no longer cautious about giving our love to our intimate partner. At moments we might beg and whimper; at other moments we might aggressively ravish our partner in love. Still at other times our loving is serene and sweet. But whether shouting, screaming, pleading, pushing, pulling, biting, or hugging, we are gifting our partner with our uninhibited and free love, flowing directly from our sexual essence without fear or doubt. If we have grown into the practice of Intimate Communion, the imaginary videotape does not pose a dilemma since we understand that the fundamental difference between rape and ravishment is simple: love. Is love the motive of every squeeze, shriek, and nibble, regardless of how forceful, aggressive, or passionate? Or is it a motive of need—the need for sex, the need for power, the need for control? Most importantly, in the practice of Intimate Communion we learn that love is something you do, not something you fall into or out of. Love is something that you practice, like playing tennis or the violin, not something you happen to feel or not. If you are waiting to feel love, in passionate sex or safe conversation, you are making a mistake. Love is an action that you do—and when you do it, you feel it. When you are loving, others find you lovable. Love is an action you can practice. Therefore, in Intimate Communion we learn to practice loving, even when we feel hurt, rejected, or resistant. First we practice love, and then our native sexual essence blooms, naturally, inevitably, because we are learning to give from our core, which includes the root of our sexuality.
   Article is adapted from *Intimate Communion* by David Deida

How the Feminine Grows by David Deida
   An essential Feminine principle is that of opening to love. The Feminine nurtures, gives life, and dances in sensual joy—although sometimes Feminine energy is also wild, fierce, or chaotic. The Feminine shines with radiance, or can appear dark and mysterious. The Feminine is the force of life altogether: the healing force of nature, the life-giving force of earth, as well as the force of destruction which re-absorbs that to which it has given birth.
   The Feminine force is not goal-oriented and directional, so the Feminine

heroine is not a warrior who cuts through obstacles. Rather, She is a goddess who opens doors with love. A Masculine warrior slices through impediments to freedom and truth; a Feminine goddess shines with love's radiance, opening passageways to the heart.

The Masculine is primarily struggling with Himself, moving beyond His own fears and learning to master the unknown terrain. The Feminine is primarily moved by Her need for love. She is also yearning for a way to release the love in Her heart.

Her whole life is about opening and loving, giving love and receiving love. Her primary suffering, and Her primary joy, is in love relationships, usually with an intimate partner, but also with Her children, Her friends, or with God.

The Masculine is essentially alone, until He is dissolved in free consciousness. The Feminine is essentially in the play of relationship, until She is dissolved in free love. The Masculine warrior wields his sword of truth. The Feminine goddess dances in the garden of love.

Just as the *first-stage* man is always looking for a bigger sword, the first-stage woman is always hoping for more love—to give and to receive. When her intimate relationship is not working, she thinks it might be her fault. Maybe she isn't giving enough love. Maybe she is expecting too much. Maybe she needs to give it another chance.

Love is her motive, and the first-stage woman will do anything for it. She will give up her own needs, her own power, her own authority. She will give them up to her children, her husband, or her teacher, in her desire for what she thinks is love. If love brushes her life, she opens to it, and out flows her energy and attention to the object of her loving. She finds it difficult to own her own needs, her own power, her own identity, because she so readily opens her boundaries in the hope of love.

Abandoning her own center, the first-stage woman seeks to fill herself with an imitation of real love. To fill her vacant heart she eats ice-cream, chocolate, and cookies. Perhaps she watches soap operas or reads romance novels.

True love seems always out of her reach: "Maybe I don't deserve love." She settles for anything that offers the potential for love: "Maybe in this relationship, there is a chance. Even though he abuses me, I think he could change. I just want him to say that he loves me."

Eventually, her pain becomes too great. She will no longer do anything in exchange for the potential of love. She will not give up her personal identity and her personal needs. Even though she wants an intimate relationship, she is determined to stand her ground. This is the *second-stage* woman, the woman who, temporarily, focuses on loving herself.

The second-stage man is devoted to self-improvement rather than acquisition; the second-stage woman is devoted to loving herself rather than to giving up her own needs—supposedly for the sake of another—in the hope of receiving love. The second-stage woman is no longer dependent on the love of another, just as the second-stage man is no longer dependent on things and people outside of himself.

The second-stage woman stands whole, frequently in the company of other second-stage women. She is no longer needy of men. In order to free herself from a Dependence Relationship with a man, she cultivates her own internal Masculine energy. She learns to assert her needs clearly, to direct herself with her own guiding hand, to see herself through her own loving eyes instead of through the eyes of an external lover. She is her own person. She has taken responsibility for herself.

The Feminist voice is one voice of the second-stage woman, celebrating her free womanhood with her sisters. As a cultural shift, women who had been following men's directions have learned to depend on their own internal voice and sense of direction. They no longer merely follow a man's lead; they allow themselves to be leaders. Such women have not only liberated themselves from men but from their own self-doubt.

Just like their second-stage male counterparts, second-stage women are independent, self-responsible, and dedicated to internal and external transformation. In fact, it is at the second-stage that men and women are most alike. They are both dedicated to self-responsibility. They are both interested in self-definition and respecting personal boundaries. They both, therefore, want to create a 50/50 Relationship.

The words "surrender" and "sacrifice" raise their hackles, second-stage women and men alike. The second-stage is all about personal power, self-authenticity, and making one's stand as an individual—worthy, strong, and not dependent. The second-stage woman and man speak loudly: I follow no doctrine, I am my own woman/man/person.

Because whole personhood is so important to second-stage men and women, they often attempt to balance their internal sexual energies. The man cultivates his inner Feminine energies and the woman cultivates her inner Masculine energies. The man may grow his hair longer, wear an earring, speak softly, smile a lot, express his feelings, and be cautious not to assert his opinion too strongly: "Whatever." The woman may cut her hair, wear less sexy clothes, use less make-up, travel widely, and speak with confidence.

50/50 Relationships are often uniquely lukewarm between second-stage men and women. Why? Because although mutual self-responsibility is a lot more whole than mutual dependency, it is a lot less passionate than mutual abandon in love.

Mutual self-responsibility, by itself, makes for a boring intimate relationship. It makes for a good friendship, which is a step up from a good slave-ship. Yet it does not allow for the full incarnation of the Masculine and Feminine forces as two magnetic poles.

Second-stage men are often afraid to love their women freely. For instance, a second-stage man often listens, becoming dull and inattentive, as his woman talks to him. He may have no real interest in what she is saying, but he feels he should listen, or at least try.

WWW.ITSNOTWEIRDANYMORE.COM

Yet, her real desire is for a deep connection in love, not for a passive audience. He can choose to give her love directly, passionately, with no hesitation: "Enough talk. I love you." Second-stage men are so devoted to their inner balance that they are afraid to sweep a woman off her feet with the kind of uncompromising love that could fill her deepest desire for intimacy.

A second-stage woman, on the other hand, is often so cautious of losing her center that she is afraid to love a man freely. She doesn't trust that he will honor and appreciate her openness. She is afraid to give a man the kind of devotional love that wants to overflow from her heart. Both the second-stage man and woman are cautious not to let go of their own boundaries or to trespass beyond the emotional boundaries of their partner. They are "safe" men and women.

How does a woman grow from the second to the *third stage*? Just as a second-stage man may come to realize that he still feels incomplete and unfinished [see *How the Masculine Grows*], a second-stage woman may come to realize she is still searching for love. Her heart is still yearning. She still feels a void, whether she is in a mutually self-responsible 50/50 Relationship or not. For most women, sisterhood is not enough, and a second-stage man is safe but not sufficient to pierce the deepest caverns of her heart.

Just as the second-stage man is reduced to zero in the abyss of absolute futility, the second-stage woman is reduced to zero in the black hole of her deep need. At the very center of her life something is missing. Her independent strength does not fill the emptiness inside her, nor does her 50/50 Relationship.

What can she do, when neither relationship nor aloneness fills the need in her heart? She must let go of her relationship and her independent stance, both, and be sucked through the black hole of her need before she can emerge like a butterfly with wings of love. When the second-stage woman dies, the third-stage woman is born. The third-stage woman no longer searches for love, but rather breathes love, relaxes in love, and radiates love.

The third-stage man lets go of everything for the sake of true freedom, and the third-stage woman lets go of everything for the sake of true love. She is no longer dependent on external love. She is no longer relying on her self-love. Rather, she is love incarnate.

Her mood is not needy, nor proud, but devotional. Her hand is not clinging, nor holding off, but blessing. She does not love like a "wife" should. She does not love like a "person" should. She loves; she is not fearful, nor cautious, but abandoned in love.

In a Dependence Relationship, a first-stage woman *seduces* a man, body to body. In a 50/50 Relationship, a second-stage woman *interests* a man, mind to mind. In the practice of Intimate Communion, a third-stage woman *enchants* a man, heart to heart. In Intimate Communion, attraction includes the mind, but quickly the mind disappears in love. In Intimate Communion, attraction is expressed through the body, but quickly the body becomes transparent in radiant energy.

LAURA LEGERE

The third-stage woman is not shy about her enchanting power of Feminine love; nor is she careful to maintain her personal identity. She knows that she is love, and so she practices giving love, moment to moment, in the ecstasy of surrender. This is the practice of the third-stage woman: to give love, to be of the disposition, "I love you," since love is her true nature.

The first-stage woman is her man's woman. The second-stage woman is her own woman. The third-stage woman is love, in the form of woman. Her identity is not derived from her man, nor from herself. Her need for self-identity is virtually gone, so bright is the shine of her love.

She wanted this unending love from a man, and no man could give her what she wanted. She wanted this unending love from herself, and she couldn't give herself enough love to fulfill herself perfectly. Now, she has sacrificed her search for love because she has gained the knowledge of love. She feels deeply, at her core, that she is love. She knows that she is either *being* love and *giving* love, or she is collapsing.

The third-stage woman knows there is no ultimate relationship to seek, no perfect self-acceptance to achieve. She understands that she will never receive enough love from a relationship nor from her self-acceptance. But she doesn't need to anymore. She has discovered when she is in the disposition, "I love you," that her life is filled with love. She has realized that when she wants to *feel* love all she needs to do is *give* love. In fact, that is the only time she feels love—when she is loving.

Her search for love is over. She may forget love, but her remembrance is always the same: I am love, and I love you. In this present moment, she practices feeling her body being lived, her breath being breathed, and her heart being opened by the radiant love that naturally wants to flow from her heart. She allows herself to be the movement of love in this present moment. She is the dancing energy of love.

Article is adapted from *Intimate Communion*

Love and Fear by David Deida

You and I both have our excuses for not opening in love with each other. Still, both of our hearts yearn to open and commune in love. I want to make this commitment with you: I will do my best to open through my fears and truly see you, feel you, and bloom you open to God with my love. Will you meet me in this commitment? Will you promise to open and give your love's offering as best as you can, even when you are afraid or hurt? If we can each commit to opening, there is no limit to how deeply our love can grow or how fully our gifts may flower. Your secret sexual desire is to be ravished, lovingly forced open in unbearable pleasure, and taken fully open to God by a man of deep spiritual wisdom, strength, humor, sensitivity, and integrity. But your past relationships probably fell short of your deepest desire for a man's loving, and your current relationship is probably also lacking. Why? The love that is deep in your heart is probably buried under layers of frustration and pain. How did these layers harden around the open yearning of your heart?

Since you were a young woman, you have probably dreamed of being lovingly taken by a good man, a man who could truly know you and cherish your heart, a man of deep integrity, a man you could trust with your life—a man you could trust to take you open into love's deepest bliss. Even now, you probably yearn to be taken by a man who truly sees your deepest heart's bright love and really knows your body, staying in touch with your unique energy as it moves and changes. Sometimes—perhaps rarely—your lover can be so present with you that your fears relax and your body opens. In these magic moments, you and your lover connect so deeply that your hearts merge as one. All separation dissolves. Your body is given over to him, and his tender strength opens you further than you can control. You may weep and tremble in his arms, beneath his body, held in his love, pressed open by the force of his true desire for your deepest heart. These moments are special, and few. Eventually, your man probably betrays you, either because he desires another woman more than you or because his love becomes shallow, his sexual neediness disgusting. Even in moments of intimacy, he doesn't touch your deepest heart or even try. You know he can love you open, perhaps more than any man ever has, and yet, over time, he becomes less interested in communing with your deepest heart. He drifts into his career, focusing on his projects, sitting in front of the TV, or satisfying his need for superficial sexual release.

So you begin to learn to live with your hurt and take care of yourself. If you can't depend on a man's love, then you can only depend on yourself. You learn to take control of your life, to guide yourself to your own destination. But something is still missing, no matter how successful your career or how comfortable your life is. You still yearn to be taken by a man's real love, to be truly seen and opened by your lover's penetrating gaze, touch, and profound heart-desire. Secretly, you still yearn to surrender to a man who is worthy of your trust. But you have not met him—and worse, you have learned that when you surrender open and give yourself completely to a man, you eventually get hurt. In the rare moments when your depth is invited, your pain comes up first and you often end up scaring your man away. So, you begin to doubt love. You lose trust in men. You surround your wounded heart with shells of emotional protection, hopefully preventing more hurt.

Your body develops tensions and even diseases after years of not surrendering, not receiving deep love, not giving yourself entirely, as you so long to do with every cell of your being. There is always tension—the tension of not being met and really stretched open in the fullness of the love you are. So when a man feels you, he feels your shells. In your face, he sees the strain of long hours or years of holding your life together while your deepest heart would rather have surrendered open in ecstatic trust. In your gait, he feels the stress of un-offered bodily devotion, while your deep heart would rather have been a slave to love, commanded open by love's torrential flow, undulated by love's boundless pleasure. Around your heart, he senses the "do not trespass" warning, and so he holds himself back from entering your life deeply. Few men are capable of entering a woman's heart and opening her body to God's bliss, but few women are capable of offering their heart and body to be claimed open in this way.

Fear is the feeling of refusal. Fear is the feeling of mistrust. Fear is the heart's contraction that withdraws openness behind walls of protection. Fear is the act of un-love, the negation of love, the refusal to open and offer love's openness as your gift. Anything less than a life of total loving is fear. Fear—the refusal to open as love—is the only reason your sexual life and relationship are less than God-blissful. Fear forms shells around your heart and closes your body so that love cannot move deeply into you, claiming you, opening you, allowing you to trust deeper than your sense of self. If you trusted and received love more deeply, you would naturally surrender open, alive as the most powerful force in the world: the devotional offering of love. Men are terrified of a woman's depth of love and the energy that moves as a woman's sexuality and emotions. And, at the same time, men want nothing more in this life than to merge completely with a woman's devotional love and wild energy.

Only as a man outgrows his fear can he handle a woman's tremendous love-energy without running. And only such a man is worthy of your devotional offering in a committed intimacy. Most men can't meet you fully. So, though your heart and body yearn to be ravished by real love, you bury your heart's longing under a life of busyness, family, friends, and distractions. You learn to plod on and get things done. You learn to seal off from your own longing. You occupy yourself with chores and to-do lists. You focus on your financial goals, or perhaps you decide to give your life to serving a social cause or following a spiritual path. You spend time with your friends, enjoy travel, exercise and take care of yourself. And still, your heart yearns, whether you are alone or with a man who is not deeply claiming your heart. Just as you have chosen to guard your heart for fear of being hurt, the man you attract will have chosen to claim life more shallowly than his true depth. He drifts uncommitted to total love because he is afraid of losing what seems like his freedom. Your relationship won't work because his freedom is false and your love is hidden; you are both afraid. You are unwilling to offer yourself completely without protection, so you attract a man without the capacity or willingness to claim you completely.

A commitment to love requires opening beyond these fears. Your lover's willingness to inhabit your life as his own, to feel your heart deeply and claim you open to love's deepest bliss, must grow—just as your willingness must grow to offer your life and heart as love, even though you know you will be hurt and betrayed in the future.

Even if you don't have a lover in your life or if your lover doesn't seem able to meet your heart with his full loving presence, you can learn to keep your heart open to the flow of love. Your heart may hurt, your heart may yearn for a deeper way to give and receive love with your man, but your heart-practice is to relax open, breathing and feeling in connection with your lover and all beings. At heart, everybody wants only to give and receive love. You can practice keeping your heart open for the sake of love's fullness, even when your man hurts you, even when you are alone, even when the pain and yearning in your heart feel overwhelming. For the sake of love's fullest flow, you can allow your heart to yearn open, deeply receiving and offering love without closing down to protect itself. Then, your life is moved not so much by your man's needs nor by your own needs of self-reliance, but by the deep wisdom-flow of love, which is alive as you and at the heart of all beings. You are fulfilled neither by a man's attention nor by taking care of yourself, but by opening as love, feeling the heart of everyone, offering your heart open so love can move you as it will, offering your life as a gift of love to all, including your chosen man. All the moments of your life—making a business deal, caring for your children, arguing with your lover—can be a dance of love's emergence, an opportunity for opening your heart and offering your life to flow open as love's wisdom, love's power, and love's indestructible vulnerability. To live with an open heart and body moved by love is your only option if you want to fulfill your deepest desire—to receive and give love's most full bliss—with or without a man.

Article adapted from *Dear Lover - A Woman's Guide to Enjoying Love's Deepest Bliss*

What Men Wish Women Knew by David Deida
A Man's Desire Grows In Three Stages

What do men wish women knew? That depends on the kind of man. We'll look at the three stages men grow through as they evolve spiritually as lovers. At each stage, men want something different from women.

1. "My way or the highway." You may recognize this attitude, or maybe your man has actually said these words to you. Some men want a woman to be obedient, and that's that. We'll call this kind of man a "me-man," because his priority is getting his own way, being king of the castle.
2. "Let's share our feelings and be fair." When a man grows beyond his need to dominate a relationship, then he is careful to divide the pie evenly. He agrees to do the dishes on Monday, Wednesday, and Friday and you agree to do them on Tuesday, Thursday, and Saturday. He takes the children to school in the morning, and you pick them up in the afternoon. We'll call this kind of man a "50/50 man" because his priorities include equality, independence, and sharing.
3. "Let's open our hearts, surrender to love, and give our deepest gifts." When a man grows beyond his need to be in charge and his need to create safety, then he has become a "heart-true man." The priority in his life is no longer about self-centered achievement. Nor is his priority to create a comfortable home and a relationship centered on fairness. Instead, like an artist learning to open and express his deepest heart, his priority is to live as love and give

his deepest gift. He wants to be with a woman who is willing to surrender, as he has, to the force of divine or sacred love. And this kind of openness can be risky business.

Sex

1. A me-man wants a woman to know how to give him physical pleasure whenever he wants it.
2. A 50/50 man wants a woman to know how to share her emotions with him, talk with him during sex, tell him what she likes and doesn't like, and express her sexual desires freely. He wants to give her pleasure as much as he wants to receive pleasure. He wants to be careful so they both feel comfortable.
3. A heart-true man's priority is not to give and receive physical pleasure or emotional comfort, but to dissolve with his lover in the ecstasy of unbounded love. He wants her body and heart to open so wide that he is drawn into her love, and through her love, into an openness of love without bounds. He wants to let go of his sense of separation and meld with his woman, opening with her as one radiant heart of bliss. In this vulnerable, unprotected embrace, he wants to consciously ravish his woman with so much love that she has no choice—that they have no choice—but to surrender open as infinite love.

Dependence, Independence, and Communion

1. A me-man wants a woman to depend on him, emotionally and financially, so he can feel good about himself and enjoy a strong sense of self-worth. Likewise, his woman wants to feel special, depended on for the pleasure, affection, and love that she gives her man. This is the least mature form of relationship, in which lovers are co-dependent, craving to be appreciated and seen as strong or beautiful in the eyes of the other.
2. A 50/50 man wants a woman who is independent and can stand on her own two feet. He doesn't want to always be responsible for her, emotionally or financially, but expects her to be able to take care of herself. He wants "space" to live his own life, and he is more than happy to give her space to live hers. This results in a modern, 50/50 style of relationship, in which two independent people share a life together out of choice rather than neediness. Although better than a relationship of co-dependence or abuse, this 50/50 relationship soon begins to feel shallow and empty of passion, almost like a business relationship, although it is fair and safe.
3. A heart-true man doesn't want a woman who depends on him. He also doesn't want a woman who stands separate, heart-guarded, and independent. He wants a woman who has grown enough to surrender her boundaries of safety, allowing her heart to open and be absolutely ravished to its depth by love—sexually and in everyday life. Although she can easily stand by herself, her heart yearns for more than the self-sufficiency she has achieved. Her enjoyment of heart-oneness is greater than her need for heart-safety. Her

bliss in communion is greater than her need for deliberate communication. Her living art is to be free, surrendered open as her true power, the flow of infinite love. Dependent neediness and independent self-responsibility were only stages on the way to this utter heart-fullness. She no longer needs a man's love, and she no longer needs to give herself love, because now she is learning to open and live as love. She is learning to breathe love with every breath and offer love through every gesture. No longer waiting for a White Knight or her own success to save her, her artful practice is to live as a blessing force of love, with or without her man.

Criticism
1. A me-man doesn't like to be criticized. No matter what he is doing, he wants his woman's support. Even if she has a good idea, he can't receive it unless he convinces himself that it was his idea.
2. A 50/50 man respects his woman's ideas and gives them as much weight as his own. If they disagree about something, he is very willing to meet her halfway. This often results in a mutual compromise, so that neither partner lives true to their deepest heart desire, but at least they honor each other's opinions.
3. A heart-true man knows that his life feels shallow unless he acts in alignment with his deepest purpose. He cherishes his woman's criticism—he realizes that in many ways her intuition is far deeper than his own— but in the end he takes full responsibility for his decisions. If his woman suggests something that changes his perspective, then he makes a new decision. But he never compromises his heart's deepest truth in order to please his woman or "go along" with her. He knows that if he gives up his heart's true decision to follow his woman's, then he will blame her if she is wrong and feel disempowered if she is right, having denied himself the opportunity to act from his deep heart and grow from his mistakes. By listening carefully to his woman and then taking total responsibility for his actions, he is free to offer her love unencumbered by resentment.

The Masculine Mission
1. A me-man uses his woman to fill the voids of his life. When he is not working, watching TV, playing golf, or reading the newspaper, he is willing to "tolerate" his woman enough to get what he needs from her.
2. A 50/50 man is willing to spend time shopping and chatting with his woman, just as she is willing to watch football games and violent action movies with him. Sometimes he listens to her talking even though he is bored and uninterested. After all, he wants to be fair, and what she has to say is every bit as important as what he has to say. He is careful to set aside his current project and spend enough time with his woman so she doesn't complain, even though deep down he may begin to resent her for distracting him from his sense of purpose.

3.   A heart-true man's priority is to open in love and give his deepest gift, just as he wants his woman to do, too. He doesn't require that she sit through a violent movie if she has to close her heart to handle it, and he doesn't want to be required to sit through a conversation if he has to fake his interest. Rather than blab about the day, there are times when he would rather sit in silence and gaze deeply into his woman's eyes, or touch her with tenderness, or ravish her with loving passion. A heart-true man wants to be with his woman without distraction, closure, or impatience. He spends his workday acting in alignment with his deepest purpose—financial, artistic, political, or spiritual—so that when he is with his woman he can offer his love undividedly and completely; he is with her wholeheartedly. She can receive his total presence, and he can receive her abundant radiance. He wants his woman to understand that even though she may be the most important person in his life, his life's mission is not necessarily centered around, nor dependent on, their relationship.

Feminine Radiance
1.   A me-man wants to be nurtured by mommy and seduced by a vixen, so he expects his woman to cook, clean, and look sexy. To him, feminine radiance means nice cleavage, tight pants, and an alluring smile.
2.   ‚A 50/50 man wants his woman to share equally in all responsibilities. He'll share with the cooking and cleaning as long as she carries her weight financially. He wants his lover to wield her masculine directionality while she smiles her feminine shine. He wants her to stay on schedule, meet her goals, and say exactly what she means while at the same time looking relaxed and radiant. She wonders, "How can he expect me to be an accountant, a word-warrior, and a goddess, all at the same time?" He wonders, "Why can't a woman be more like a man?"
3.   A heart-true man may do business with his woman, but he acknowledges that he isn't with her for that reason; nor is he with her only for love, which he freely enjoys with his friends and entire family. He has *uniquely* chosen his woman to be his most intimate feminine source, the only person with whom he opens in full sexual expression and gifting. A heart-true man understands that the most glorious feminine radiance is a gift borne of open heart, relaxed body, and fulfilled soul. Therefore, he does his best to create a sanctuary in which his woman's love can bloom through a trusting heart, a blissful body, and a soul entered by his deep presence. Even if she is a corporate CEO, in their intimate time together he honors her deepest feminine desire, which is to open in love so fully, to surrender in trust so completely, that she is filled by the divine bliss that flows from her heart's deepest chambers. He wants to open and surrender with her, so that her radiance bathes his life in glory as his presence swoons her naked soul in divine delight.

The Bottom Line

1. A me-man wants his woman to know how to bolster his self-image and plea-surize his body.

2. A 50/50 man wants his woman to know how to communicate clearly, stand independently, and be half-and-half, willing to change the car's oil or remove the dead mouse from the trap and then wear lace and silk to bed.

3. A heart-true man wants his woman to know how to give her soul's deepest gifts, and how to open her heart and body with him in a surrendered merger of unprotected fullness so they flow freely with, and dissolve in, the boundless love that is their heart's deepest desire.

Deviations of the Feminine Heart by David Deida

Just as the Masculine in each of us seeks perfect freedom through progressively more enlightened ways of "dying" to Himself, or of releasing Himself, the Feminine in each of us seeks perfect love through progressively more enlightened ways of "surrendering" Herself. The Feminine wants to open Herself and be filled with love. Thus, stage by stage, the Feminine may find Herself surrendering to, and hoping to be filled by, intimate partners, family, food, social causes, and God. When the Masculine has truly released His self-focus and the Feminine has truly surrendered Her self-protection, then true Intimate Communion is possible. Communion is surrender to the point of oneness. Communion is un-guarding your heart and welcoming a free flow of love, until all sense of difference has melted and your sense of separate self has disappeared in the fullness of love. Like true Masculine ego death, true Feminine surrender is also a form of liberation, a form of dying to resistance, a form of yielding into love, so that all refusal has been rested in the deep surrender to love itself.

Intimate Communion for both men and women is union with, in, and as love. The Feminine first seeks love by surrendering Herself to various people or activi-ties. She surrenders to Her family, to Her lover, to Her friends, to Her teacher, to Her own desires, to a career, or perhaps to a form of therapy or religion. Because She doesn't understand Her heart's primary impulse, the Feminine tends to devi-ate from true and ultimate fulfillment—whole bodily surrender into inherently fulfilling love-communion—by surrendering to people and activities which are far less than fulfilling. In a first-stage moment, the Feminine might even hope to fill Herself with love by surrendering to abuse. Charlene, a client of mine, would come for a session every week. And every week Charlene would tell me how her lover would yell at her for hours, criticizing and belittling her, even beating her, slapping her face, and sometimes throwing her across the room. Within a few hours or a few days, he would apologize and they would make passionate love. Everything would be OK for a while, and then the cycle of abuse, violence, and making up would begin again.

I have counseled as many women who remain in abusive relationships as I have men who continue to be angry and violent. Aside from the co-dependent fears of losing their partner, these women and men experience a deviated form of satisfaction throughout the cycles of abuse and passionate sex. He continues to release himself through his fits of violence and orgasm, and she continues to surrender herself to the strong presence of his physical dominance and sexual aggression. Although they may feel guilty, hurt, and confused, a part of them enjoys this drama. Part of him feels emptied of tension via release, and part of her feels open to and filled by love via surrender.

When understood from the point of view of the Feminine's primary heart-impulse, this form of deviance can be seen as an unhealthy approximation of loving self-sacrifice. For the Feminine, any form of giving Herself up to the Masculine force is an approximation of surrender. Although it is a far cry from being sweetly ravished and overwhelmed by love in the ultimate embrace of perfect Intimate Communion with a partner, it is still a form of surrendering to another in the hope of fulfillment, just as is raising a family, opening sexually with Her lover, or giving Her time and energy to a social or religious cause. In each case, She hopes to be filled with love by surrendering Her sense of self to something else. In the case of a woman in a Dependence Relationship like Charlene, this "something else" is often the control or aggression of her man. If Charlene were able to re-connect with her primal impulse, the impulse to be deeply surrendered to and overwhelmed by love itself, then she would be able to pull herself out of the deviance she has entered. She would be able to cease surrendering to the aggressive force of her angry man, re-gather her energy, and follow her primal impulse to give and receive true love more and more deeply.

As Charlene becomes less dependent on her abusive relationship, she will grow naturally toward a 50/50 Relationship. When she is finally able to stand independent and free of her abusive relationship, however, Charlene will probably notice a strange sense of loss. Intellectually, she knows that she is better off letting go of the abusive relationship. But, emotionally, she feels something is missing. In a strange way, in a way she may be reluctant to admit even to herself, she misses the feeling of fulfillment that her old relationship did provide—she misses the sense of surrender and love, which was at least an approximation of her heart's true desire. It was the deepest love her heart knew. Of course, she shouldn't go back to her abusive Dependence Relationship. That would be taking a step backward. Nor should she remain forever on guard against surrender, since the only way to fulfill her core desire is to lose her fearful resistance and allow herself to be overwhelmed in the knowledge of love. Rather, she should become integrated by balancing her internal Masculine and Feminine and strengthening herself, growing out of her Dependence Relationship and toward a 50/50 Relationship, should she choose to be in any relationship at all.

In a second-stage moment of internal balance and integration, the Feminine is more independent, strong, and self-assured than in a first-stage moment. However, the second-stage Feminine has Her own way of deviating from the primary impulse at Her sexual core, the impulse to be surrendered whole bodily in the blissful, ravishing, overwhelming force of real love. Many second-stage women deviate from the primary impulse of their heart into an apparently safer course of surrendering to a career or to a social or spiritual ideal. They know better than to surrender to a man—they have already suffered this form of surrender in a Dependence Relationship, and they have been hurt. So, a second-stage woman may refuse to surrender in intimacy at all, holding herself separate and well-guarded for the rest of her life. Or, she may surrender halfway, into a 50/50 Relationship, and continue to seek the pleasures of greater surrender through other, less risky means. She may seek fulfillment by surrendering herself into her career, her therapy, her social cause, her religion, or her creative art.

For example, it would be very natural for Charlene, after leaving her abusive Dependence Relationship, to seek fulfillment by losing herself in her career, going to a therapist, or joining a weekly support group of some kind. She would then surrender not to a man's anger, but to her daily professional schedule and her work of self-integration. As a second-stage woman, she would tend to deviate from her basic impulse by attempting to achieve fulfillment through devoting herself to herself: to her work, her creativity, and her personal growth.

The modern world is filled with men and women like this, men and women who are driving around and around in the cul-de-sac they originally discovered in the hope of achieving fulfillment. The second-stage Masculine in each of us drives around and around searching for His approximation of a death-like sense of release through epicurean sexing, through knowledge, or through creative accomplishment. The second-stage Feminine in each of us circles through Her friendships, Her career, Her artistic creations, and Her intimacies, as if Her heart would be truly fulfilled, someday, through these means. Throughout this search for fulfillment, She is careful to remain independent, to stand Her own ground, and especially not to surrender too much to an intimate partner.

If the second-stage Feminine clings to Her position of independence too long, however, She will suffer the loss of deep emotional and sexual loving. Why? Because the pleasure of being ravished in love is precisely negated by holding too tightly to one's own ground. Eventually, the second-stage Feminine realizes that, try as She might, whether dependent or independent, She can't seem to get enough love. However satisfied She is with Her career and Her friendships, She still feels an emptiness in Her heart that yearns to be filled, a sense of loneliness that yearns to be touched.

By recognizing our second-stage obsession with career, creativity, therapy, or religion as a deviance, we can re-gather our energy and align our life with our basic impulse—the impulse for limitless freedom, ecstatic love, and boundless happiness. If you have a Feminine sexual essence, then the texture of your impulse will probably feel like a desire to be overwhelmed by love, to be surrendered into love. Therefore, rather than surrendering yourself so much into your career, for instance, you must learn to take a portion of your energy and devote it to surrendering directly into love—not to a lover, not to a therapist, not to your creativity, but to the force of love itself, which lies latent in your heart.

LAURA LEGERE

By making this shift in how you devote your energy, you grow from a second-stage orientation and a 50/50 Relationship into the third-stage practice of Intimate Communion. You begin to truly embody your heart's desire, directly in each moment. You understand that you have been deviating from your primary impulse by making the mistake of assuming that you would be fulfilled by giving your energy to your family, to a lover, to a career, or to a creative endeavor. In the practice of Intimate Communion, you begin to give your energy to the expansion of your heart, directly. More and more, you rest in the real knowledge of love.

Article is adapted from *Intimate Communion*

Orgasmic Love by David Deida

Before I understood how to open with you, I tried giving you orgasms so I knew I was a good lover. But now, all I want is your surrender. I want your heart's pleasure to ripple through your open body and saturate my life with your love. Your body's openness to love's flow draws me into you, and through your heart's surrender I am opened to the love that lives as the universe. Whether you have an orgasm or not while we make love, your body's trust and devotional openness is my secret doorway to love's deepest bliss. Your body's openness—your capacity to surrender open with your whole body so your heart can be ravished and taken by love—is a doorway to ecstatic spiritual depth, with or without a man. If your body can't open, your heart can't shine. When your body is surrendering open with pleasure from deep within, then you can open and offer your heart fully from the inside out.

Orgasm is one form of sexual pleasure. You may never have had what you call an orgasm, or you may have had many. It doesn't really matter. What matters is that your body can open in love's blissful surrender. If your pelvis is locked and your vagina is closed down or numb, then your heart is prevented from offering love fully through your body. Opening through orgasmic surrender, alone or with a lover, can provide a unique opportunity to offer your deepest love and uninhibited yearning through your fully expressed body.

Clitoral Orgasms. You may or may not have a man in your life, but for now, imagine that you are in bed with your lover. He strokes your belly and caresses your breasts. He touches you gently inside your thighs, trailing his fingertips from knee to crotch. Fondling, touching, loving, he eventually kisses you between your legs. With sensitivity and skill, he licks, nibbles, and sucks your most sensitive flesh, while also touching your feet and legs and belly and breasts with his hands. Your breath becomes shorter and faster. Your eyes close. You grab his hair and push his face tightly against you. Breathing rapidly, an orgasm seizes through your body, your voice high-pitched, shrieking, your face tense, your body tightening, and then relaxing, after one or two or three clitoral orgasms. These orgasms do require emotional or spiritual trust with your partner—self-stimulation or a vibrator can be used to achieve this pleasure without a partner. Clitoral orgasms can prepare you for surrendering open more deeply. Vaginal or G-Spot Orgasms. You have been making love for almost an hour, your lover thrusting in and out, his body pressing against yours, while kissing you, biting your neck, and pinning you beneath him with his loving strength. "Don't stop," you groan, as your body relaxes open. Your arms spread out from your sides, your heart opens, your mouth opens. Your moans are long and deep from your belly. As the waves begin, your sound goes deeper. You gaze into your lover's eyes, moist with vulnerable affection, your bodies softening into each other, your hearts melding. You take him in more deeply, opening your body to him, giving yourself to him, yielding fully. You gush between your legs, your vagina grabbing him, milking him, pulling him in more deeply. His constant rhythmic loving sends a purr through your body like a cat vibrating. You relax more deeply open, and waves of open pleasure begin radiating from your vagina out through your whole body. Like an ocean of openness, your pleasure draws him in deeper. You offer your heart to him, unprotected. Your soft bodies press together, your hips moving in uncontrollable waves, your mouth ohh-ing in open pleasure, your body surrendering layer after layer more open than you have in a long time. The G-Spot, an area of spongy tissue a few inches inside the anterior or front part of the vagina, is very sensitive in many women. If you are capable of experiencing G-Spot orgasms, but haven't yet, this tissue can hold much tension, anger, and pain. This area of your vagina can be massaged according to your verbal guidance—slower, harder, softer, faster—eventually relaxing you enough to open in deep orgasmic waves, possibly even ejaculating fluids from this spongy tissue.

Cervical Orgasms. Your cervix is the physical source of extraordinarily deep orgasms. As with your G-Spot, your cervix may be quite sensitive and painful to the touch if you haven't regularly allowed full pleasure to move through your cervical area. But with a few weeks of receiving massage near your cervix, this area opens. And if you have a man in your life, then when you make love, as your lover's thrust stimulates and opens your cervical area, your emotional and spiritual surrender can lead to tremendous orgasmic revelations of love's bliss.

After an hour of heart-connected, passionate, sexual merger, imagine that your loving together with your man continues. His entrance into your body is deep, persistent, creative, unyielding. His strong hands hold your wrists, his belly presses deeply down into yours, his gentle force enters you again and again, opening you, opening places you have never felt to open. You feel utterly claimed, taken open to God, obliterated in his deep loving. You let go even more deeply, dying in the intensity of his loving, crying as all love bursts you open. You are killed by bliss, softly, sweetly pervaded by his tender love. Your skin dissolves. Your edges melt. And again, even deeper, you let go of something you didn't know you were holding, a minute clench deep in your heart opens, giving open to him, to God, and your tears flow. Forgetting beginning and end, your orgasm opens deeper and deeper. Layers of surrender are offered up through your depths, out through your body, as he penetrates you to gone. Together, you open as such deep love all disappears in the fullness of bliss, light melting all hold, love filling all space, an unbearable fullness surrendering open endlessly, boundlessly, abundantly, no place remaining unopened, untouched, unrevealed. Your orgasm unfolds and unfolds as never before, love rippling you open, your face drenched in tears, your body in sweat, bright beyond form. You are being breathed open in blissful death, ravished open, unable to hold on, surrendered open by a force you are so deeply, the living light of love that you always almost knew now shines so fully, wracking you open in unbearable pleasure, your deepest womb grasping and letting go, seizing and releasing, the pulse of the universe opening out from deep between your legs, opening out from deep within your belly, your heart given open fully, all of you given, offered in utter devotional surrender. For days, love's bliss flows freely through your body. Your motions are full of grace, your face shining, smooth, and radiant with love's flow. Your lover and your friends can feel this orgasm's openness continuing to resound through your gestures, the way you walk, the expression in your eyes, the relaxed tone of your voice, surrendering you open for a long time after the sexual occasion has ended. Surrendering open to the fullest flow of pleasure can be an important part of opening fully and offering your deepest love to the world and to your man if you are in a relationship.

With practice and skill, solo or with a partner, your orgasmic capacity deepens along with other aspects of your capacity to offer your deepest heart. Over time, you may experience deep orgasms without any sexual stimulation at all, simply while dancing, or doing yoga, or breathing fully and offering yourself open to God to take. Your body is built to be opened by love and to open as love's offering. Love is who you are, and love is the gift you are born to give. With practice, you can learn to live open as devotional fullness, as if you were receiving deep sexual ravishment and offering your heart's fullest gifts through your whole body. How would you be breathing right now, sitting right now, moving right now, if your body were being entered by a man of enormous love and integrity, a man who felt so deeply into your heart that you were forced to reveal your most subtle closure, taking you open so exquisitely you could hardly bear to open in so much love and trust?

To live open, your body can practice feeling sexually open, whether or not you are having a physical orgasm or even having sex. Through sex and in everyday life, you can practice feeling, breathing, and offering yourself open as if the passionate force of a divine lover were entering you sexually, opening your heart and body as wide as the universe shines.

Adapted from *Dear Lover - A Woman's Guide to Enjoying Love's Deepest Bliss*

David Deida

Acknowledged as one of the most insightful and provocative spiritual teachers of our time, best-selling author David Deida continues to revolutionize the way that men and women grow spiritually and sexually.

Known internationally for his unique workshops on spiritual growth and sacred intimacy, Deida has designed and developed a remarkably effective program of transformative practices that addresses spiritual awakening in mind, body, and heart. He is a founding associate of Integral Institute and has taught and conducted research at the University of California Medical School in San Diego; University of California; Santa Cruz; San Jose State University; Lexington Institute, Boston; and Ecole Polytechnique in Paris, France.

His teaching and writing on a radically practical spirituality for our time have been hailed as among the most original and authentic contributions to personal and spiritual growth currently available. Deida is known worldwide as the author of hundreds of essays, audiotapes, videotapes, articles, and books that bring to light an integral approach to spirituality. His books include the best-selling underground classic, *The Way of the Superior Man*; several practical texts on authentic sexual spirituality, including *Finding God Through Sex, Blue Truth*; and the autobiographical novel about highly unconventional spiritual training, *Wild Nights*.

Sacred Sex

Margot Anand is an internationally acclaimed authority on Tantra, bestselling author, and much-beloved teacher and founder of "SkyDancing Tantra." Margot's books, videos, CDs, and DVDs are widely regarded as the seminal teachings for integrating spirituality and sexuality. Her popular books are available in numerous languages, and include *The Art of Everyday Ecstasy*, *The Art of Sexual Ecstasy*, *The Art of Sexual Magic*, *Sexual Ecstasy: The Art of Orgasm*, and *The Sexual Ecstasy Workbook: The Path Of SkyDancing Tantra*. Her DVD, *The Art of Orgasm*, which presents the MORE session, and her three-disc DVD trilogy, *Margot Anand's The Secret Keys to the Ultimate Love Life*, inspire a whole new generation of lovers as well as offer a refresher with some fun new twists to longtime students of her classic methods.

Steve & Lokita Carter, founders of The Institute of Ecstatic Living, are licensed SkyDancing Tantra teachers and empowered by Margot Anand as her principle lineage holders in the USA. They have been practicing, educating, and living their powerful teachings for many years as well as instructing the world-renowned "SkyDancing Tantra Love & Ecstasy Training" exclusively since 2003.

They delight in sharing with each other and through their workshops what they have learned over many years of ecstatic living and the tantric lifestyle as a married couple. When they joined together their love and variety of talents, they emerged as a powerful, fun, dynamic, and loving teaching team.

Steve and Lokita are the producers of the best-selling tantra DVDs, *Tantric Massage for Lovers, The Breath of Tantric Love, Tantric Yoga for Lovers, Chakra Wisdom: An Active Meditation for Clarity, Insight & Transformation*, and have appeared on radio and TV stations across the United States and most recently on Discovery Channel.

VitalzymeX

World Nutrition's VitalzymeX can help…
* To reduce inflammation

With a potent blend of systemic enzymes that includes the powerful anti-inflammatory qualities of serrapeptase and a highly active form of the enzyme protease, VitalzymeX is the most effective natural therapy to reduce inflammation and related pain. Its lack of toxicity makes VitalzymeX the ideal alternative to the non-steroidal anti-inflammatory drugs (NSAIDs) thought by many to be at the root of more serious health concerns.*

* To remove scar tissue and excess fibrin in the blood

VitalzymeX is the one preparation with the ability to reduce both inflammation and scar tissue/fibrosis. Its highly fibrinolytic enzymes lyse (eat away) at the scar tissue that can limit mobility and diminish the functions of other organs. These enzymes also help to improve circulation and reduce the clots formed by excess fibrin in the blood.

* To modulate immune function

Systemic enzymes have proven helpful in the treatment of autoimmune conditions by eating the antibodies the body creates to attack its own tissues. If the immune system is too low, systemic enzymes help to increase immune function by boosting the efficacy of infection-fighting white blood cells.

WarriorSage

The Path of The **WarriorSage** is for those who want their personal and spiritual growth fast, and without the "fluff" of New Age thinking. It is for you if you are willing to do what it takes to really make a huge difference in your life, and eventually in the lives of those you love, and beyond that even to serving the world open with your Awakened WarriorSage heart, skills, and insights.

The Warrior within You is that part of you that faces, feels, and moves through your fears with courage, openness, honesty, humility, and heart, and does whatever it takes, despite obstacles, to realize your goals.

The Sage within you is that part of you that, with one foot in the world and one foot in the mystery, is able to play, laugh, and love through life.

The WarriorSage within you is that part of you that lives with the intention, courage, action, and endurance of the Warrior combined fluidly with the humor, transcendence, wisdom, and love of the Sage.

WWW.ITSNOTWEIRDANYMORE.COM

All you have to do is take the first step and make the commitment to participate full-on at one of our Sex, Passion and Enlightenment Introductory workshops.

Here you will get firsthand, in-your-body experience of how to live with passion, how to realize enlightenment, how to make it all work for you on a practical day-to-day basis, as well as get a good foundation to propel you to your fullest potential... Mind, Body and Spirit! *www.ItsNotAnymoreWeird.com*

Sex, Passion & Enlightenment introductory workshop is an introduction to living from your deepest spiritual sexual essence. It is about expressing your full Masculine or Feminine Essence and is based on the revolutionary work of one of Satyen's teachers, David Deida.

Satyen Raja's purpose is to awaken as many people as possible, in the time he has in this world, to their full potential and to help them integrate and sustain this level of enlightened practice.

As a student and adult he devoted himself to seek out the best and the brightest of teachers, practices, and trainings he could find, designed to grow beyond his own limitations. He scoured the world, training with the most profound teachers, who gifted him with their deepest knowledge, wisdom, and teachings.

His goal is to give you what works—what really works in real time. Everything he teaches on The Path of the WarriorSage is time-proven in the real world by thousands of his students. He will share with you only proven strategies, teachings, and practices that are guaranteed to help you realize your deepest spiritual happiness fast!

He sees so many people walking half-asleep, their deepest expression of themselves lying dormant deep inside, locked behind thick walls of complacency, apathy, and resignation. His purpose is to evoke you out of your slumber and shake, rattle, and roll you (lovingly, of course) to realize you can have a much more fulfilling life than you can possibly imagine!

He is here to let you know there is a way you can melt your barriers quickly, safely, and have a great time while you're at it!

Real spiritual growth takes dedication, tenacity, courage, vulnerability, and heart, and I want you to know YOU HAVE ALL THAT IN YOU! It just needs to be awakened!

The Wholefood Farmacy

"The thousands of vitamins, minerals and phytochemicals [beneficial plant compounds] in whole foods act synergistically together to create a more powerful effect than the sum of their parts, producing a result which cannot be recreated by supplements," says Jeff Prince, vice president for education at the American Institute for Cancer Research.

The Wholefood Farmacy makes eating healthy easy, convenient, and affordable. They offer pure, nutrient-dense, ready-to-eat, whole food meals, snacks, soups, smoothie mixes, and treats for the children. All of the foods are vegetarian; most are raw and vegan as well. The Farmacy also offers many gluten-free and nut-free whole food choices for those with food sensitivities.

Even when people have sufficient knowledge about nutrition and health, the supply of healthy food products is often inconvenient and/or unavailable. The Wholefood Farmacy makes convenient organic whole food meals and snacks that help you eat healthy wherever you are.

Try the Wholefood Farmacy's "Phi Plus" (A complete blend of 45 delicious organic raw whole food ingredients)

Dates, rolled oats, Thompson raisins, sesame seeds, sunflower seeds, almonds, cashews, hazel nuts, pecans, walnuts, brazil nuts, prunes, grape seed oil, pure salt, figs, raspberries granules, grape seed oil, walnut oil, brown rice flour, quinoa, amaranth, barley, flaxseed, millet, rye, oat flour, banana powder, green peas, pumpkin seeds, orange powder, blueberry powder, nutritional yeast, peach powder, guava powder, ginger, cinnamon, aloe vera powder, clove, strawberry, coconut, lemon oil, orange oil, stevia leaf powder.

Yoga

Home Yoga's mission is to create a safe, nurturing, and supportive environment for all individuals to explore the practice of yoga. We strive to encourage and support students in building confidence and knowledge of this ancient practice with experienced and loving teachers. Our goal is to assist in helping all students in taking their practice from our HOME to theirs.

Terri Dyer is the owner of Home Yoga and has been practicing yogic philosophy most of her adult life. She started her physical yoga practice in 1998 as a way to express her deep love of life. Through asana (yogic postures) she found a way to bring the song and dance of her mind, body, and spirit together as one complete symphony.

She completed the 8 Limbs Teacher Training in January of 2004 and continues to study and be inspired by many teachers, including Shiva Rea, Ana Forrest, Seane Corne, and Rodney Yee to name just a few.

Terri's classes tend to be physically challenging, which allows students to find their power from within. She teaches flow (vinyasa) linking breath to movement, integrating strength through grace, alignment through insight, and wisdom through contemplation and meditation. Classes focus on breath work, creating heat from within, core strengthening, creating space in the hips and shoulders, opening the heart through backbends, and looking at the world with a new perspective with the help of inversions. She encourages students to challenge themselves with enthusiasm.

Kitty Wittkower is one of Home Yoga's advanced teachers and her training focuses on asana technique, with a special emphasis on therapeutics, for injury and illness.

Kitty has practiced yoga since the early 1980s and in 1992 was certified in the Iyengar method. Recently completing another teacher training, with Shiva Rea in Seattle in 2005, she continues her education with other yoga luminaries that include: Dona Holleman, Dharma Mitra, Ana Forrest, Sharon Gannon, David Life, Gary Kraftstow, Kathleen Hunt, and most recently Les Leventhal.

There are a variety of teachers to choose from who can fit your style, from the beginner to the advanced.

Young Living Essential Oils

The Missing Link
Gary Young on Essential Oils

The following is a transcript of "The Missing Link," a very informative and interesting talk on essential oils given by Gary Young, founder of Young Living Essential Oils. It is lengthy and full of powerful information. Enjoy.

Welcome to Young Living Essential Oils and the world of aromatherapy. Aromatherapy may be a new term to many of you listening, but it is an ancient art and science which began its re-entry into the modern world only a few years ago. With a biblical foundation and historical information from different cultures around the world, there is much that we have to learn and study.

We at Young Living are very excited to share this life-changing information with those who are looking for new truth that might bring healing of different dimensions resulting in untold health, happiness, and prosperity.

Young Living Essential Oils came into existence through Gary Young, a very unusual and visionary man who, through the most amazing circumstances, finds himself teaching seminars, formulating in his laboratory, plowing the fields on his tractor, designing and building equipment for the farm operations, training his horses to pull a plow, and running a multimillion-dollar business.

He grew up in the mountains of central Idaho with no electricity or running water, where he and his brothers and sisters were taught by their parents how to live from the earth.

At age 24, a terrible accident left him paralyzed for life. Rejecting the medical diagnosis, he began his search for natural ways to heal his body. He studied the sciences of hematology, medicine, anesthesiology, acupuncture, pathology, nutrition, herbology, and many other types of healing modalities. With great determination, 13 years later, he ran a half-marathon and finished 60th out of 970 participants.

LAURA LEGERE

After receiving a master's in nutrition and a doctorate in naturopathy, he opened a family practice in Chula Vista, California, and a research clinic in Mexico where he could do research in the areas of natural healing. His work in Mexico was of such magnitude that in 1985 he received the Humanitarian Award from the State Medical Examiner's Office of Baja, California (one of only six ever awarded) for his research and successful treatment of degenerative disease. It was in this clinic where he was introduced to essential oils, which started him in the direction that he continues today.

In November of 1995 Gary was invited to speak at the UNIDO (United Nations Industrial Development Organization) International Congress on Essential Oils held in Eskisehir, Turkey. He presented research that is being conducted on the Young Living Blends and Single oils at Weber State University and on organic farming and plant germination at the farm in Idaho. His work was received with tremendous enthusiasm and many who attended showed great interest in what we are doing as a means for improving their economics.

Gary loves the challenge of research and discovery, which has driven him deep into the history of early medicine and essential oils. He goes from the ruins of ancient Egypt to the archaeology archives of the Hebrew University in Jerusalem to the British Museum Library in London to his own laboratory and now, today, to the chemistry department at Weber State University to prove the validity of this ancient science. It is an exciting adventure for those who love the discovery of truth.

Gary Young is a man of great faith and belief in God, who loves his home and his family and whose greatest joy is being of service to his fellowmen and, perhaps in a small way, helping them to realize their dreams. Gary is one of the foremost authorities on essential oils in North America. So now, let's join Gary Young in one of his lectures and see what we can learn about this most fascinating subject.

Gary Young:
Essential Oils, just to give you a real simple analogy…if we were to take the plant and human body and put them side by side we could do some very interesting comparisons. You see, in the human body we have a substance called blood, and that blood has a very specific purpose. That purpose is to transport nutrients to the cells, to nurture and feed the cells. One of the primary agents in the blood that is responsible for the delivery of the nutrients through the cell walls is called oxygen. If we take the oxygen out of the blood what happens? We would die very quickly. The cells begin to mutate and give off a toxic gas that creates a host for disease, and today we live in an environment where we are deprived of oxygen because of the air we breathe, the food we eat, and the water we drink. Because of that we have set ourselves up to be victims, and it's quite obvious by

what's going on in our world today. When we look at Essential Oils, they have the same role, and play the same function in the plant, as the blood does in the human body. The Essential Oil is the blood of the plant.

How many of you have cut your finger? What happens? You bleed. Why do you bleed? (Audience: to cleanse) Exactly, to cleanse and to kill the bacteria because you have to do that to start the regeneration process of the tissue. Okay, how many of you ladies have seen a leaf on one of your houseplants torn or damaged? What comes out? It's a liquid, isn't it? It's called the resin by some, some call it the blood of the plant. Some call it the life force of the plant but it's the same thing, it bleeds. It bleeds to cleanse that part where the plant is damaged, to kill the bacteria. You see, the Essential Oil is like the blood, it's a transporter system, and the primary ingredient inside that oil is called oxygen.

It has been discovered and determined now through research and the translation of the papyrus and hieroglyphics in Egypt that oils were the first medicine of man. Even before herbs were used, oils were extracted from the plant and used before the actual plant was used. As of three years ago, it was documented that Essential Oils produce the highest level of oxygenating molecules of ANY SUBSTANCE KNOWN TO MAN. So when we think about that, that we can get actual oxygen from the oil, it's quite exciting. Now not only can we get oxygen from the oils, but we also get negative ions and we get ozone. Are they important to us? (Audience: yes) Why? Can bacteria live in ozone? Can bacteria live in a negative ion environment? No. You know it's interesting when you look at what's going on in our world, because there's a big wave that has hit the United States called antioxidants. Right? Everyone's looking for antioxidants and antimicrobial substances to take.

We're just going to walk through some things real quickly and show you why Essential Oils are the missing link in our health field today and why everyone and every home needs to have them.

Let's look at what the human body is up against today. We look at what's causing the poisons that we're inhaling, the industrial contamination that's affecting our air. Look at the foods we're eating today, fried foods in grease that causes carcinogenic activity in the blood. Foods that are devaluated and therefore we get no enzymes from the foods that we're eating. The foods that are coming from the fields are sprayed with chemicals. The ground is saturated with chemicals and has been for over 50 years…and we wonder why we can't get good wholesome food today. Not to mention the environmental contamination that's going into the aquifer, along with all of the contamination in the entire food chain that the human body is subject to. We absorb this not only through the food and the water but through the pores of our skin and the oxygen we breathe in through our lungs.

These chemicals go down into the intestinal tract and cause a weakening of the membrane wall and they leach through into the liver and cause cell mutation. It changes the pH chemistry of the blood and all of a sudden we've got a problem.

We start creating a host for disease and then we wonder how can this possibly happen? So detoxification is extremely important today in our lives.

It's really interesting to know that Essential Oils, because of their structure, will literally push chemicals and metallics out of the cells. How? Because they have the highest level of oxygenating activity of any substance known to man. Oxygen pushes toxins out and pulls potassium back into the cell. Essential Oils will re-establish normal cell function and balance.

Time magazine, the September 12th issue, I'm sure most of you have seen it: "New Virus and Drug Resistant Bacteria are Reversing Human Victories over Infectious Diseases." How can this happen if we have a healthy body? Can we have infection if we are healthy? Can we have cancer if we're healthy? Can we have AIDS if we're healthy? No, of course not. So let's be realistic and look at it.

This was quite interesting because if we look down here at the bottom it says: "More than 850 people have come down with cholera in Southern Russia and officials fear that disease could erupt into an epidemic." While this article was being published and they were talking about 850 people in Russia, they never even made mention of the thousands of people they were digging holes, open pits, and burying in mass graves in South America from cholera. Did anyone see that on CNN? We need to start paying attention and waking up to what's going on around us.

Look at this: "Some microbes can reproduce in just 20 minutes." And this article goes on to talk about how the drug makers are fighting back, and yet how every time they produce a drug, the bacteria or the virus mutates and develops its own immunity to the antibiotic. Now that's quite interesting because when you know these things are fact, and then when you come to understand oils, and realize that at this point in time, today, they have not found ONE virus, that can create an immunity against an Essential Oil.

Look here: "The question ceases to be when will disease be gone?" This is interesting then we look at the statistics: "Respiratory infections bacterial and viral: 4 million deaths, diarrhea and diseases related, viral and bacterial: 3 million deaths" this is per year "Tuberculosis bacterial," now we have a new VIRAL tuberculosis, do we not? They don't even mention the viral tuberculosis here, just the "bacterial" million.

Hepatitis B virus: 3 million. Protozoa, malaria: 1 million. Measles, viral 880 thousand. Tetanus, 600 thousand. AIDS, viral 550 thousand. They don't even talk about cancer and heart disease. We're just talking about diseases related to virus and bacteria, yet they don't even list the new tuberculosis virus, or the new Hanta virus, the flesh-eating virus, the streptococci A, the Ebola virus. You know, there's so much going on that we're not even aware of what's happening.

I think many of us also have a tendency to want to ignore it, we don't want to deal with the truth. Why? We don't know what to do about it, true or false? Okay, look here: "Where will the next deadly virus appear?" Then it goes on to talk about the agents, small pox, AIDS, hepatitis B. How many of you are familiar with the Ebola virus and the symptomatology of it? Are you aware that Ebola virus causes decomposing of the internal organs and the smooth muscle tissue inside the human body? And once a victim contracts the Ebola virus, three to five days and they're dead? Do you know what happened in Wanamingo, Minnesota just last week? Where eight people died from what they're calling the new streptococci virus that causes people to die in three to five days, their tissue and internal organs degenerated? It was the Ebola virus but they're saying it's the new streptococci A. An epidemic. This is interesting: "The price of doing nothing will be millions of lives." And it's happened before. Look here: "Killer flu 1918-1919, killed 20 million people." So we're not dealing with something that just popped into our world today. There have been viruses around since the beginning of time. Look at what happened during Moses' time. Look at the 16th century plague in England and Europe that claimed millions of lives. Why is it happening? Why do we have more of it today? Because we have a weaker immune system. How are we going to build it?

Okay, what are we going to do about these things? Look at this article here in the March issue of *Readers Digest*: "The invisible invaders. The question is no longer when will infectious disease be wiped out, rather it is where will the next new deadly plague appear." You need to read it because this article talks about how with every antibiotic that they have made, the viruses mutate, the bacteria mutate and create their own immunity against the antibiotic.

We need to read these things so we're aware of what's going on, and be prepared. Let's look at some of the things that cause it. "Water suspected in illness. U.S. health official speculates that local water sickened hundreds of AIDS patients during the spring. Groups warn of risk of drinking water." "New TB a time bomb." This is *USA Today* news cover story. We need to be aware. "Flu on tap. Milwaukee blames illness on tap water. Tainted water blamed for unlike illnesses," it just goes on wherever we look. "A contagious fascination with infections as lethal viruses make news the public ponders what if, the hot zone?" How many of you have seen the movie *The Outbreak*? Well, that's not just a movie, that's a reality. "Ancient ills return with a vengeance." Viruses that they can't kill, they can't control.

Now I want to spend time showing you what's exciting. This comes right out of the Cairo University research department, Dr. Radwan S. Farag who is our colleague in research at Cairo. I worked with him for three years. "Safety evaluation of Thyme and Clove Essential Oils as natural antioxidants." If we're going to fight something let's fight with what God gave us to fight with. Look here: "antimicrobial activity of some Egyptian spice Essential Oils," hard copy research. We're not just here to talk about folklore medicine. "Antimicrobial action of Essential Oils. The antimicrobial action is probably the one property of Essential Oils that has been known for the longest time." Isn't that interesting? But do you know about it? Do you read about it? Do you get to hear about it in the US of A? Of course not.

How many of you know someone who has diabetes? Let me show you what's going on at Cairo University with diabetes, they CURE it. Look here, this is just one of the simple studies that was conducted on diabetes. Blood glucose levels, this was control group with insulin right here. Then they used bitter fennel and it dropped it from over 275 to 200. Common dill oil, below 200. Coriander brought it down to normal range. Simple Essential Oils. Yes, they're correcting diseases in many places in the world. Look what came off the Associated Press two months ago, very interesting. "Scientists examine role of food derivatives in preventing cancer." Is anyone interested in cancer prevention? Cancer regression? Well, look at here: "Soybeans, lavender oil, and orange peel" and we jump over here: "Cancer fighting powers of plant oils. Small quantities of lavender have been shown to work against breast cancer in lab animals." In animal studies these say we've got both the prevention of cancer and the regression of cancer. How many would sooner have chemotherapy than a bottle of lavender oil?

Now this is something that's very exciting. We need oxygenation, antioxidants, and increased frequency. What's a frequency? Is frequency important to us? Are our bodies electrical? Absolutely. And it's very interesting when we study this and see that not only is our body electrical but everything around us has an electrical frequency. But there's different types of frequencies and this is what's interesting. Because your lights overhead, they also have a frequency called 60 hertz. Essential Oils have a frequency from 52 to 320 hertz. But the difference between the oil frequency and your light frequency, television, telephone or microwave, your electrical AC frequencies are incoherent, chaotic frequencies. They fracture the human electrical field. Essential Oils have a coherent, harmonic DC frequency, so they're harmonious with the electrical field of the human body. So Essential Oils give us oxygen, antioxidants, and frequency.

Now, I make food supplementation and was the first to create this type of formulation, the first to develop it in the world and that is using Essential Oils in the food supplements. Why? Because we found Essential Oils work as a transport mechanism in the food supplements. The reason we're starving to death nutritionally is because we're not assimilating the nutrients on the cellular level. Essential Oils have the ability because they're soluble with the lipids in the membrane to go through the cellular wall, and to carry with it nutrients that there's an association with. Because that's their purpose in the plant life, to transport nutrients through the cell wall and deliver it inside the plant. So when we took Essential Oils and put them inside the plant it was very exciting, because we got a delivery system.

Now I want to back up a bit and give you something to think about. Going back to the blood, the blood is the transporter of nutrients. Vitamins, minerals, proteins, amino acids, hormones, enzymes. That's the pathway they travel to go to the cells. Then the cell wall has to be receptive to those nutrients and those health food ingredients. But when we have a deficiency in oxygen, the cell membrane literally will start to thicken because the pH changes, and when it thickens, then the oxygen that's present there, also being compromised because of lifestyles, is not able to get the nutrients through the wall, and so we wind up with the nutrients in the blood serum but we can't get it inside the cell, and so we wind up having the cell mutation, creating a host for viruses, bacteria, and germs. Now, if Essential Oils are responsible for the oxygenating molecules, they are antiviral, antifungal, antibacterial, and immuno-stimulating (which I'm going to show you in a minute, hard copy from the medical research), and they have the ability to transport nutrients, that they are the life force of the plant, what do you suppose happens to that oil when we cut the plant and dehydrate it? We evaporate 98% of that live substance that's responsible for the healing force of that plant.

As I look through the audience I see quite a few people here that are probably old enough to remember the days when they used to gather herbs fresh in the pasture or field or out on the hill, and come home and make up their poultices and their teas and their extracts, and it worked. So you tell your children about it and when your children get sick they go down to the health food store and buy a bottle of that same herb in a capsule form, take it home, take six bottles of it, and nothing happens. And we wonder why? It is because modern man has taken the life force out of the herbs by dehydration. So when I discovered that, or learned about that, that's when I started spraying the oils back into the powdered herb and it brought back the bio-availability of the nutrients that weren't there before or available to us before, because the catalyst agent had been evaporated out of them. So we were the first to put Essential Oils back into the plant, and re-establish that activity.

If we want to cleanse our body, we want regeneration, and we want immunity, then we've got to start working on self inside out, and outside in. It's really beautiful because we can create that simply by putting oils on the body.

Now look at lemon oil. Lemon oil is pressed from the rind or the peeling. Now this is taken right out of my French medical encyclopedia, this is hard copy research, this is not my work and of course you can see that it's in French, Latin, and so what we're looking at here where it says "active principles" these are the constituents or the chemical ingredients found inside of lemon oil that are identifiable. Many have not been identified yet. We look right here, there's one agent here called sesquiterpenes. I'm going to talk a little bit about it as I go along. Sesquiterpenes. The reason that's important is because they just found in 1994 at the Medical University of Berlin, Germany and Vienna, Austria that sesquiterpenes go beyond the blood-brain barrier. Now, I don't know how important that is to anyone, but I'll fill you in.

It was stated by the Medical Association, October of 1993, that if we: "could find an agent that would go beyond the blood-brain barrier, we could treat MS, Parkinson's, Lou Gehrig's, and Alzheimer's successfully." June 1994 it was documented that the agent of sesquiterpenes has the ability to go beyond the blood-brain barrier and was discovered in high levels in frankincense and sandal-wood oils. I attended a three-day medical conference in Grasse, France September

LAURA LEGERE

5th, 6th, and 7th of 1994. I saw this research presented, and I saw the brain scan slices of before and after the inhalation of frankincense and sandalwood and how it increased the oxygen production in the limbic system, particularly around the pineal and pituitary glands, and increased the secretion of antibodies, endorphins, and neurotransmitters. Documented hard copy from Berlin and Vienna, Austria.

Let's look at lemon oil: "Anti-infectious, antibacterial, streptococci bacterial, antiseptic bacterial, antiviral" this is how the doctors prescribe lemon oil to be used in the hospitals in Europe. There are 150 hospitals in England alone now prescribing and using Essential Oils for treatment. "Respiratory infections, liver insufficiency in children, digestion insufficiency, insomnia, phlebitis, thrombosis" and they use it as a disinfectant in the air and the cabinetry and medical cabinets and in hospitals throughout Europe. And what do we use in America to disinfect with? Drugs.

Lavender, this is another beautiful oil. Now I showed you from the Associated Press about lavender, did I not? Look at this one here, this is lavender again, and look at the profile that we see, and there's sesquiterpenes, okay? Now not only are sesquiterpenes and terpenes able to go beyond the blood-brain barrier but they also have been found along with phenols and cineols to contain the highest level of oxygenating molecules of all of the constituents in the oil. Let's look at what they say lavender will do. This is out of Paris, France, incidentally.

We have: "Antispasmodic, decongestant, muscle decontraction, hypotensive, anti-inflammatory, anti-infectious, staph, cardiotonic, anticoagulant of fluids." And of course they prescribe it for the spasms in the solar plexus, insomnia, dermatosis, infections, allergies. How many of you have taken allergy shots in your life? Isn't that bizarre, to know that lavender is used for allergies, in fact what was discovered two years ago is that you take lavender oil, and incidentally it has to be pure lavender oil, this doesn't mean you can just run down to the health food store and buy any old lavender oil that's sold on the market because you see, in America people don't understand Essential Oils, but what they do understand is marketing. They know how to buy the garbage that's rejected from France, and bring it to the United States and cut it with propylene glycol, and synthetic constituents like linalyl acetate, and put it in a bottle and sell it as Essential Oil of lavender, and if you don't know the difference, you're just a victim. So if you go down to a health food store and you see a half ounce of lavender oil on the shelf for $5-$8 a half ounce, you KNOW that you're getting garbage, because pure lavender oil, you can't buy it in France for that price. So those are things that are very important.

Just to give you an understanding, there are four hybrids of lavenders, but they're called lavandins. They're not therapeutic for aromatherapy use, but that's what's sold in the United States predominantly, because people here don't know the difference. Our lavender we produce in France, because we have our own farm in France and we have our own farm out in Idaho. We do our own growing in order to produce top quality. You have to distill this plant and that's how the oil is extracted, through steam distillation. It has to be at low pressure, low temperature, and lavender has to be in the chamber for a minimum of one and a half hours, better two hours. But the commercial distilling in Europe for the perfume industry distill lavender oil in fifteen minutes at 400 degrees and up to 150 pounds of pressure, and they pump chemicals into the water while they're doing it. So these are things that are very important for you to know. It's not just a matter of running out to a health food store and buying oils because the people who are marketing oils predominantly are in it for the money, they don't care about the purity and they haven't taken the time to study.

I've spent 11 years in Europe, Israel, and Egypt studying the history and working in the universities. My studies have been in the Medical University of Geneva, Switzerland. I started in 1984. The University of Paris. I have worked in two hospitals in Paris. I've studied in the Warwick University, the London University, the University of Cairo where I've spent three years working, studying, and traveling. The Hebrew University in Jerusalem. It's been an incredible study. I've spent five years off and on in Southern France learning the ancient art of distillation so we can maintain that purity.

Now let me share with you some of the things that just came out of the Warwick University that I brought back last year on lavender oil. This is really exciting. Lavender, a native of the Mediterranean region, France is a major producer. Now Idaho is going to take over. "A fragrance component of pharmaceuticals, antiseptic ointments, creams, lotions, cosmetics, including soaps, detergents, creams, lotions and perfumes. Lavender waters and colognes. However, lavender now is starting to be widely used in aromatherapy for the treatment of burns, scalds, inflammation, wounds, ulcers, eczema, dermatitis, fainting, headaches, migraines, influenza, insomnia, hysteria, tension, infection, asthma, rheumatism, and arthritis." Now when you can get a bottle of lavender oil for $15, who would want to have aspirin?

This is interesting, these are just the constituents responsible for all that activity in Lavender oil. This is just a small portion. It's interesting to see when we look at the linalyl acetate level right here, we're at a 441. That's a relatively good quality oil. The lavender oil we're producing at the farm in Idaho has a linalyl acetate level of 67. The highest quality produced in the world. Look at here, "Toxicity: subcutaneous injection showed low toxicity, no human phototoxicity reported." So it's totally safe, and that's the beautiful part of Essential Oils. You don't have to be concerned about having side effects from pure oils. Cut, adulterated, synthetic...absolutely, but not pure, not the way God intended it to be.

Why is it valuable? How do we get oils quickly into the system? Through the olfactory nerve, to the pineal, pituitary, amygdala. When you breathe an oil into the system, and through the nasal cavity, it is first picked up by the neurons that hang down from the olfactory, right between the eyes at the top of the sinus cavity. Those oil molecules are carried within milliseconds into the center of the brain. Now they have found that through the inhalation of Essential Oils into the mid-brain system, they will cause a secretion of antibodies instantly, endorphins and neurotransmitters. Now we're seeing a direct response on the immune system from the inhalation, and topical application of Essential Oils like none other that has ever been created. So diffusing puts the oils into the atmosphere in your home. You're getting increased oxygen because it releases the oxygenating molecules, you're getting increased ozone and negative ions because that's where it comes from in nature, from the plant oils. You're getting the antiviral, antibacterial, antifungal, germicidal properties and the immuno-stimulating. You're inhaling this. In fact I just got a copy, a hard copy in on the Internet just last week from Alester University in Northern Ireland where they did a study of diffusing, vaporizing Essential Oils into an atmosphere with 210 colonies of bacteria, and it killed all 210. So it makes the most perfect air purification system that has ever been invented, or rediscovered, and we can't afford to be without it.

How do we know these things happen and how do they work? By simply studying the properties in the oil. This is thyme vulgaris, this is a chromatogram. Everybody knows what camphor is, right? It's soothing, it's penetrating to the tissues. Camphor is synthetically made from the active ingredient called camphine. So when we look at this oil, which is thyme oil, we know that it's going to have a very powerful effect in penetrating. We look at the pinenes, the germicidal, we look at the cineols here, they're antibacterial and antiviral. We look at the terpenines, they're antiviral in action. So when we take an Essential Oil in the laboratory and analyze it, we know instantly the value it has. Depending upon the percentage of activity, it will tell us whether it's a pure oil or whether there's been something done with it.

So the science is incredible. This is clary sage that we grew at our farm this past summer in Idaho. The highest linalyl activity of any clary sage, 72. Most clary sage ranges around 57. Down here you have sclerol a transoxide to sclerol. That is what converts to estriol in the human body, which produces natural estrogen. So how many of you ladies are taking some synthetic hormone? You got it right here in your plants.

When God created this world he created everything naturally for us, and he gave us every substance we will ever need to protect our bodies from all the things that we have to deal with. Just like he gave to the Israelites. Yes, they were faced with a plague, and if you saw the movie *The Ten Commandments* it depicted it as an avenging angel, a green fog that floated through the city. It was a plague. Scientists and researchers of Egypt say it was nothing different than the AIDS we have today. They're convinced of that. So what did Moses do to protect the children of Israel from that plague? He used Hyssop oil in the lamb's blood. You can read about it in Exodus, chapter 12. You can also go to Exodus chapter 30 verses 21 -27 and read about the formula, the oil formula that the Lord gave to Moses to give the children of Israel to protect them against the ravages of the diseases and the plague. We're talking about a substance that's been around since the beginning of time with a biblical foundation, and man has ignored it. It has been lost and forgotten.

Not until 1921 did it start to come back into our time, from an old gentleman, Dr. Rene-Maurice Gattefoss. He was a French cosmetic chemist working in his lab one day when there was an explosion, and he received a third-degree thermal burn on his hand, wrist, and forearm. Knowing he needed to reduce the temperature, he reached over where one of his colleagues had just set a container with liquid in it, thought it was water, plunged his hand into it, and it was lavender oil. And it healed his burn without a trace of a scar. That man was so excited that being a chemist, he took the lavender apart to understand and find out how it healed his burn without a scar. From there he gave the research to Dr. John Valnet, who was a medical doctor in Paris, France. Valnet did nothing with it until the postwar years of World War II when he was working with war victims from shrapnel wounds and losing them to gangrene because the antibiotics wouldn't work. Dr. Gattefoss sent him some oils and said, "Try the oils." He started using the oils and he saved every single patient. That was the restoration of aromatherapy as it's called today. 1946. That's how new it is, yet the studies never really started until 1967. It is the most exciting thing that we have.

Now this is just a little bit about Essential Oils' frequency. My scientific research team was the first to discover Essential Oils literally contain an electrical frequency. We did a study of over 200 subjects at the Eastern State University in Cheney Washington. We found that the average body frequency range is 62-68. The brain frequencies are 10 hertz higher than the body during the day and then it reverses during the night and the brain frequencies are 10 hertz lower, body frequencies are 10 hertz higher. We took two young men who had a 66 hertz frequency, one held coffee, his frequency dropped to 58 in 3 seconds. The other one drank it. His frequency dropped to 52 in 3 seconds. The young man that drank the coffee, we didn't let him have any oils, it took three days for it to go back up. The young man that just held the coffee, we let him breathe the Essential Oil of RC, his frequency went up in 21 seconds. We found that disease begins at 58 hertz frequency. Flu starts at 57. Candida 55. Epstein-Barr at 52 and cancer at 42. What this tells us is that when we do things in our lives that compromise our frequency in the human body, we can become a victim. Essential Oils re-establish a normal frequency in the human cells, documented at the Eastern State University.

Another thing that's really exciting is regeneration. How can you regenerate something if you can't stimulate circulation and activity? This comes right out of Dr. Richard Restick's work, top leading neurologist of the United States, Washington DC. This man helped me to discover that the oils were electrical. How? Because we discovered that hearing could be restored with the oil of helichrysum. Not only from loss of hearing but from deafness, BORN deafness. Three people now have total restoration. I went to him to ask how, he said the oils are electrical. They stimulate the firing in the axon. They increase the neurotransmitter that converts in the axon to electron, it fires across the synaptic gap right here. He said in a birth defect, the nerves didn't connect. He said that the oils will literally increase the firing of that synapses, and it will jump across the gap and connect to that nerve that did not connect. Once it starts firing it will start growing together until it hardwires. So Essential Oils have the ability to stimulate the regeneration of damaged nerve tissue. Helicrysum.

How do we use oils? Diffusing in the air, through the feet. Many of you here are probably reflexologists and are certainly working with the feet. Start working with oils through the feet.

How many of you have experienced pain and suffered with pain for days and days and days and couldn't get rid of it? You've taken pain medication, Tylenol, morphine and whatever to kill pain? How would you feel if you knew that if you broke a bone and you can take a single oil and rub it on that broken spot and stop the pain within three to six seconds? You can do it with Essential Oils. There's a formula that I made called Pan Away. It has two oils in it that are responsible greatly for that, one is helichrysum and the other is wintergreen. Wintergreen oil, like spruce oil contains methyl salicylate. It works like cortisone on the tissue and it's a topical anesthesia. Helichrysum is a topical anesthesia. It's beautiful. So I made a formula called Pan Away for that purpose.

Another way to work with oils is through the ears, auricular. How many people here have emotions? Is there anyone that has no emotional problems at all? Do you know that the ancient Egyptians used oils to do what they call cleansing of the flesh and the blood. Removing the evil deities from the mind. Because they believed if they didn't remove the evil deities from the mind, which we call negative emotions, they couldn't come back into the body they left in the tomb.

I was allowed March last year, one year ago, to go into a secret chamber where this ritual was performed, and I was allowed to photograph the walls. We started translating the hieroglyphics that told about this ritual, it was a three-day ritual, and they used oils to take the people through it and totally eradicate the negative memory and memory trauma from the people. I've started teaching and working with people with oils for eradicating emotions and emotional trauma, it is life changing. Working through the ears. In fact we have a little oil blend called Hope. If you ever feel depressed, manic depressant, or suicidal, a couple of drops and rubbed right there and it'll take it away in just a matter of seconds.

Another beautiful area to work through is through the spine. Just massaging the oils up and down the spine, getting it into the nerve meridians, to get into the organs and glands in the body. It's absolutely incredible. We had a gal in Denver, Colorado yesterday, I had a seminar there and we had over 150 people in the seminar. She had a great big large knot on her spine. We just rubbed simple oils of spruce and birch and frankincense on it and it dissolved HALF in 20 minutes. And 150 people gathered around and watched.

Okay, let's show you what's going on in the antiviral activity. We have a little kit called the Essential 7. It has lavender, peppermint, and lemon oils in it plus four blends, because I formulate blends. One of the blends in there is Pan Away that I just mentioned. Another one is called Peace Calming. I made that for people who are hyperactive like children. I made it also for hyperactive parents who have hyperactive children. I made another one called Purification to kill airborne bacteria in the home, odors, mold, fungus. It's incredible. In that packet is also one called Joy. This has rose oil in it, the highest of the frequencies, 320 hertz. It has ylang ylang in it, which balances the male/female energies. It also is a powerful support to the heart, for tachycardia and arrhythmia.

Another oil blend that I just made recently is called Immupower. Because of these new viruses and our immune system weakening I knew that we had to have something to help support that system. So I went to work studying, and I put this formula together. These oils that I'm going to present now are in that formula. This is Ravensara aromatica. It's a plant that's a combination of clove and nutmeg which grows in Madagascar. Of course you see the sesquiterpenes. Sesquiterpenes stimulate the immune system. Look at here "anti-infectious, antiviral, antibacterial" and it's indicated for aminopharyngitis, sinusitis, bronchitis, viral hepatitis, viruses of the intestinal, cholera, herpes 1 and 2, infectious mononucleosis, insomnia, muscular fatigue. That's one of the oils in Immupower.

Here's another one, this one you ladies probably have in your kitchen called oregano. You know, you need to quit cooking with it, and start juicing it and snorting it, okay (laughter). Look at here, "phenols," the number one constituent that's responsible for the oxygenating activity of oils, "anti-infectious, large spectrum of action against bacteria, virus, fungus and parasites, immuno-stimulant."

This one you'll like, Frankincense, it's talked about in the bible, the holy anointing oil, it's mentioned 52 times in the bible. Okay, "sesquiterpenes" again go beyond the blood-brain barrier. Look at here "anticatarrhal, expectorant, antitumoral, immuno-stimulant, antidepressant, bronchitis, catarrh, asthma, ulcers, cancer, immuno-deficiencies and nervous depression."

I got involved with a doctor in Scottsdale, Arizona, Dr. Terry Friedman, a medical doctor. I asked him if he would like to do some research and work with the oils to see what he could create, and he said, "I would love to." As of this day, one year from the time we started he now has nine cancer patients out of nine in remission from prostate and lymphoma and Hodgkin's. That's documented, by the way.

Hyssop oil, the oil that Moses used. Look at here, "anticatarrhal, mucolytic, decongestant, anti-inflammatory of the pulmonary, regulator of the metabolism and lipids, anti-infectious, large spectrum staphylococci, pneumonia, parasites. Prescribed for rhinopharyngitis, bronchitis, pneumonia, cystitis, post-infections, sclerosis, plaque, ovarian problems." It just goes on and on and on.

Mountain savory. Look at here, "anti-infectious, major activity as an antibacterial agent, antifungal, antiviral, antiparasitic, immuno-stimulating," and here they use if for "candida, cystitis, prostatitis and right on through arthritis, rheumatoid arthritis." That was mountain savory. All of these oils are found in the formula called Immupower.

This is cistus oil, commonly called rock rose. Beautiful oil. Same thing, here we see the phenols again, okay, "anti-infectious, antiviral, antibacterial, regulator of neuro-vegative degeneration of the nervous system, auto-immune." Also for arthritis, rheumatism, plaque and other things but primarily for viruses of the auto-immune system. What is AIDS?

Okay, we had a beautiful situation in Pottstown, Pennsylvania just a couple of weeks ago. A nurse at one of the seminars said, "Dr. Young, can I share a story with you?" and I said, "Yes." She said, "One of the doctors I work for has a patient that has lupus. She's had it for a number of years and as she is getting older the lupus has just been progressively getting worse and worse and worse. She was in the hospital for tests and change of medication and my doctor told her there was nothing that could be done. He said just to get her affairs in order." She said, "I felt so bad that when she started to leave I just walked her out and I gave her my bottle of Immupower. I said, why don't you take this home and just rub it on and see if it'll make you feel a little better and help you a little bit." She said, "Some of the oils here have been found to help support the immune system." The lady took it home. Three days later she called the nurse back and said, "What did you give me?" The nurse said, "Why?" She said, "I'm feeling better. My strength is coming up, my energy is coming up." Five days after that, which was a total of eight days, she returned to the doctor for a checkup. He could not find one symptom, not one trace of lupus. God knew we were going to have these diseases. He knew what we were going to deal with. Do you think he put us down here to be victims? Absolutely not. He gave us everything we need to take care of the human body.

This is clove oil by the way, and look at here, "anti-infection, antibacterial, large spectrum of action against gram positive and negative, antiviral, antifungal, antiparasitic, antiseptic and a general stimulant. Antitumoral, dental infections, viral hepatitis, colitis, cystitis, viruses of the nerves." What is MS? Look at here, "cancer, Hodgkin's." That was clove oil, simple clove oil. I mean it is so incredible to see what can be done and what can be created. So I have made a major focus on creating formulas to support the immune system.

It's been really a pleasure to be here and share with you what I call the missing link, and what I also find to be the most exciting thing that has been rediscovered in the world, and that's the world of Essential Oils, how we can use them in our food products, in our food supplements, and create a beautiful opportunity to build the immune system and not become a victim. Let's be thankful for what we have, let's always have thanks in our hearts for all that we have. Let's live with that and keep a smile on our face, and joy in our heart. Let's share with the world the blessings God gave us a long time ago.

Thank you for coming and participating.

End Of Transcript

Laura's note: Gary Young and Young Living Essential Oils have been the foundation for my recent healing recovery and since 1996 a tremendous gift in my life mentally, physically, and spiritually. I cannot imagine being without them. I hope my story can help you on your unique journey whatever that may be.

November 2008, update on Peter's health: His blood test showed the Hep C virus had dropped so low that Dr. Messer said it looked like the beginning of a cold; his liver count was healthy and he had physical energy he had not felt since the mid eighties. Teresa's Quantum Biofeedback Machine showed no more mercury in his system and his profuse itching had stopped. He had completely recovered from shoulder surgery he received August of 2008 to address his limited motion, pain and numbness in his right arm and hand. The surgery whittled off his enlarged shoulder bone and some sharp calcium deposits cutting into his nerves. Raindrop Therapy, VitalzymeX, NingXia Red juice and his physical therapy exercises sped up his recovery time from the surgery to two months. He is a new man. His radio show is not broadcasting at this time and may pick up again in the near future. Now he could explore himself without the low energy drain of so many health issues.

September 2009, update on my last facial reconstruction surgery. Harborview Hospital in Seattle performed a four-hour task by taking out two steel plates and nine screws around my right orbital bone, straightening my septum, and whittling down the crushed bone on the bridge of my nose. Afterward my face was completely purple and my eyes were swollen shut. Peter and my sister Ruth kept applying the essential oils throughout the day and I continued doing the same in the days that followed. The surgery was performed Thursday morning September 3rd and by Saturday September 5th the discoloration was gone and the swelling was way down. A week later the surgeons checked their handiwork and commented on how good I looked considering what had been done. They said normally anyone else would still be black and blue and more swollen. I mentioned that I used my own medicine and told them about essential oils. I looked forward to my new face forming.

Update on Peter and me. I know this may come as a surprise, but Peter and I are no longer together. As it turns out we do not have a similar foundation of what we desire in a relationship. It became so completely different that we agreed to bless each other on our separate journeys. I learned even more about myself in the last year with him. No matter how much I love someone, I will not try and stop them from making their choices that do not work for me. I am very clear about my path and love myself enough to choose not to follow someone else if it throws me off my goals, focus, and passion. I loved Peter from the deepest part of my being and am glad to have experienced loving like that and will continue to love deeply with whoever stands before me. May we all practice the freedom to love with abandon and not be attached to an outcome.

After all is said and done on this fantastical journey through thick and thin I have concluded that everyone can benefit from having a Wifey; the steadfast, tried and true relationship is with my Wifey. She still stands before me and reminds me that I am a powerful Goddess no matter how many trials and tribulations I go through.

Urban Dictionary definition of a *Wifey*: Term used to describe serious girlfriend/wife who you plan to stick around for *lifey*.